# A Stor
## for LIFE

# A Stoma is for LIFE

## A study of stoma care nurses and their patients

BARBARA WADE

DAPHNE HEALD RESEARCH UNIT
Royal College of Nursing of the UK

Wade, Barbara
  A Stoma is for LIFE: A Study of Stoma care
  nurses and their patients
  1. Gastrointestinal Surgical Stomata patients.
  Nursing
  I. Title
  610.73'677

ISBN 1-871364-06-X

Typeset, printed and bound in Great Britain by the Alden Press, Oxford

# Acknowledgements

The work of analysing, collating and writing up is one of the most pleasurable tasks in research, but a longitudinal study like this entails a great deal of effort and fieldwork. This was carried out with tireless enthusiasm by a team of researchers which included, over time, Elaine Bielby, Paul Wilson, Alwyn Moyer and Merry France Dawson. Similarly, the study entailed a great deal of secretarial work which was cheerfully undertaken by Janet Hussein.

I would particularly like to thank the Royal College of Nursing library staff, Rolf Knobel and the London University Computer Centre for their help in data analysis, and Professor Charles Clark, Robert Chapman, Keith Jacka and Tom Keighley for their comments and advice. I am especially grateful to Pauline Fraser and Shirley Allen for their help in the early stages of the study and to Martin Bland for his painstaking appraisal of the script.

This study would not have been possible without the co-operation of many nurse managers, ward sisters, stoma care nurses and surgeons who generously gave their time to set up the study and comment on the issues involved; I am grateful to them all.

The study forms part of a larger programme to evaluate the work of clinical nurse specialists. I would like to express my sincere thanks to the charitable trusts and public companies whose contributions to the Unit made this programme possible. The staff of the Daphne Heald Research Unit are very grateful to Ann Norman Butler for her fund-raising efforts on our behalf.

Finally I would like to thank those who made the biggest contribution of all: the patients themselves who shared their feelings and gave us their poems.

Barbara Wade

To

# Lady Daphne Heald

who made it all possible

# Contents

# Aims of the Study

1  To evaluate the benefits to ostomates of specialist nursing care

2  To provide information on the problems encountered by patients following stoma surgery

3  To evaluate the implications of specialist nursing posts for other members of the health care team

4  To assess the future training needs of clinical nurse specialists in stoma care.

# Introduction

This study has been specifically designed to test the assumption that provision of specialist nursing care will improve the plight of the ostomate. It is primarily patient-focused, and is based on interviews with patients in which they give their own account of the events leading up to surgery, their hospital experience and the care that they received before and after discharge. It is essential to note that these accounts are based on patients' perceptions and recollections of events. Inevitably these accounts will contain some distortion due to faulty recollection, misunderstanding or selective perception. We make no apology for this and proceed on the basis that we need to gain an understanding of these processes if we are to improve the standard of patient care.

In 1980 the DHSS estimated that there were more than 100 000 people with a permanent stoma and that approximately 5000 permanent colostomies for rectal cancer were constructed each year in NHS hospitals in England and Wales. In 1984, Fleming estimated that there were approximately 130 000 people with stomas in the UK of which approximately 40% were temporary ostomates. Figures, based on market research, suggest a more conservative figure of between 64 500 and 72 000 established stomatists, with approximately 18 450 new patients each year (Stringer, 1985). Stringer also suggests that no substantial changes in the annual number of new patients are foreseeable for the next decade. It would seem that the need for stoma care will remain as pressing as it was in 1980 when the DHSS outlined the following needs in a pamphlet entitled 'The Provision of Stoma Care':

- psychological preparation of patients and relatives before surgery when this is possible;
- a suitably sited stoma and provision of an acceptable and well-fitting appliance;
- advice on the management of the stoma, the appliance and skin care;
- advice and psychological support over problems that may arise during recovery from surgery;
- continued care and advice after discharge from hospital (e.g. in case the appliance needs to be refitted or adapted because of reduction in the size of the stoma, or in relation to changes which may also occur due to age or the onset of other illness).

This same document points out that, although the responsibility for advice to patients before and after surgery rests with the consultant and the general practitioner, the specialised functions of fitting stoma appliances and advice on adapting to an ostomy are essentially nursing functions. It was suggested that, relative to requirements in a given population, there should be a trained stoma care nurse in each health district.

Built into this document is a clear assumption that the introduction of specialist stoma nursing posts would result in an improved service to patients. It was felt that this should offset the resource implications by way of bulk purchasing and correct fitting of appliances, reductions in unnecessary changes of appliances, repeat prescriptions and length of stay in hospital. However the document also states that:

> 'It will clearly be some time before comprehensive services of this kind can be made available in all or even a majority of districts.' (p. 3)

This last statement appears to have been unfounded. In 1982, a brief survey of all health districts in England and Wales revealed that the number of nurses specialising in various aspects of patient care had more than tripled since a similar survey which had been carried out 3 years previously (Castledine, 1982). The largest single specialty was that of stoma care. In 1982 stoma care nurses were employed in 60% of districts and several others were considering such appointments.

Such a major development in nursing should not rest on an assumption that the service to patients will be improved. Indeed this assumption was challenged in 1985 with the claim that research had demonstrated no improvement for colostomates in their quality of life or access to buffer services over a decade, despite the 'pouring in' of resources into stoma care nurses and training schools (Devlin, 1985). The two studies cited in support of this claim were based on samples which were clearly disparate in terms of sex distribution, age and time since surgery. However, the challenge remains. In this specially designed longitudinal study the care received by patients in randomly selected districts which employ stoma care nurses is compared with that received by patients in other randomly selected districts.

The first chapter outlines the theoretical framework on which the study is based. The implications of stoma surgery are considered and the literature is reviewed to identify those factors that might make it easier or more difficult for patients to adapt to their changed circumstance. The stoma care nurse is one of these factors and the chapter contains a fairly detailed account of her role. The design of the study and details of the sampling procedure are outlined in Chapter 2.

Chapters 3 to 8 are based on interviews with patients 10 weeks after their surgery. These and later chapters are prefaced by patients' poems which were given to us during the interviews. The third chapter presents a profile of the patient sample, together with an account (based on patient recall) of the events leading up to surgery. Chapters 4 and 5 are concerned with patients' experiences of hospital. Chapter 4 focuses on patient information and includes sections on what patients remembered being told about their diagnosis and the reasons for surgery, and the information that they received preoperatively and postoperatively, including information on appliances and their management. The extent of patient satisfaction with information is also explored. Chapter 5 deals with patients' experiences in hospital, their length of stay, their first reaction to their stomas and learning to manage their stoma appliances.

Chapter 6 gives an account of patients' experience in the first two months following discharge from hospital and covers the formal and informal support which they received, dietary modifications they may have made, their physical state in terms of the extent and severity of physical symptoms and readmissions.

Chapter 7 covers self-care and the management of appliances. Patient satisfaction with appliances is assessed and the problems experienced by patients are both described and assessed.

Chapter 8 deals with patient adaptation, defined in terms of measures designed to assess quality of life, level of social activity and psychological adjustment.

Chapters 9 to 11 are based on interviews with a reduced sample of patients one year later. Chapter 9 presents a profile of the sample covering mortality, stoma reversal, physical symptoms at the time of interview, readmissions, problems experienced and sources of help. Chapter 10 deals with self-care and the management of appliances and covers the use of different types of stoma products, patient satisfaction and problems with appliances. Chapter 11 focuses on the quality of life, level of social activity and psychological adjustment of patients one year after surgery. Sections are included on marital relationships, holidays, returning to work and acceptance of the stoma.

In Chapter 12 the findings from the study are discussed in the context of information gained in the later interviews with staff. The limitations of the study are clearly stated and the findings relating to patient adaptation are compared with those from previous studies.

The final chapter addresses the question of the organisation of care. Information gained from the interviews with staff is used to explore the incentives and disincentives to the appointment of clinical nurse specialists. The generalist/specialist argument is re-examined in the light of both the findings of the study and the interviews with staff. Finally, a different approach to the design of a curriculum for the education of specialist nurses is suggested.

All the stoma care nurses who were involved in this study were female. In order to distinguish between patients and nurses the female gender is used when referring to stoma care nurses and the male gender is more commonly used when referring to patients.

Many of the ward sisters we spoke to said that they had no idea what happened to their patients after they were discharged from hospital. It is hoped that the study will fill this gap and that it will appeal to all nurses who may come into contact with patients who have had stoma surgery.

# 1

# A Framework for Evaluation

The role components and associated tasks of the stoma care nurse will be described later in this chapter. These were taken from the many papers written by stoma care nurses and, as we will see, there are gaps in this literature. For example, the importance of preoperative preparation has been emphasised many times, but what happens when patients are admitted for emergency surgery? Is there any attempt to compensate the patient in some way for the lack of preoperative preparation? In seeking to evaluate the possible benefits to patients from specialist nursing care, it is important to identify other factors, such as an emergency admission, which may also have a bearing on patient outcome. The thoughts outlined in this chapter provide the framework which will be used as a basis for later analyses. As a first step in deriving this framework it is necessary to consider the implications of stoma surgery.

## The implications of stoma surgery

It may be supposed that many patients experience stress on admission to hospital. The sources of stress have been described by Cohen and Lazarus (1982). Some of the 'threats' that they outline are particularly relevant for patients who undergo stoma surgery. For example, the threat to body integrity and comfort, including bodily injury and permanent physical change, is particularly relevant for ostomates and is additional to the physical pain which all surgical patients may experience to some degree. Similarly, other sources of stress for ostomates arise from the loss of autonomy and control and the need to alter their self image. Together with these concerns, ostomates may face uncertainty about the future course of their illness and doubt about resuming their customary life-style. All these aspects of stress are described by Kelly (1985) who kept a diary of his experiences and his perception of events before and after stoma surgery.

### Change in body image

Many of the articles written by stoma care nurses deal with the stress induced by a change in body image. This stress is, perhaps, epitomised by patients' reactions when they see their stoma for the first time. It is often difficult to get patients to look at their stoma and many are surprised or shocked when they first see it (Cunningham, 1969; Morrow, 1976). Very many patients describe an unpleasant initial reaction no matter how well prepared they have been (Druss et al, 1968, 1969). Kelly (1985) states:

> 'The protruding stoma and its attachments looked horrible. Moreover, I now realized how uncontrollable it was and what being permanently incontinent implied.' (p. 521)

The reasons underlying the initial feeling of mutilation, shame, degradation, horror and subsequent fear of rejection described in the literature have been attributed to child-rearing practices (Donaldson, 1976) and to concepts of 'normality' (Eardley, 1979).

Barney (1978) suggests that the sudden change in body image, experienced by ostomates, always gives rise to anxiety and that bodily distortion is expressed as a distortion in the total self. Thus it would seem that the change in body image leads to a change in the self-image overall. In other words, it gives rise to confusion and a negative change in the way an individual perceives himself. This change will be greater for those whose self-esteem was initially unrealistically high, or for those who have always taken a great pride in their appearance. In this respect, whereas the formation of a stoma is grossly disfiguring to the body, it is probably more disfiguring to the mind (McKenna, 1979). Indeed, it has even been suggested that the violation of body intactness may be perceived, on a fantasy level, as physical or sexual assault (Orbach and Tallent, 1965).

## Loss of control

Children are taught from an early age that uncontrolled elimination is dirty and unacceptable (Reeves, 1984). The gaining of control over elimination is a means of gaining love and support from parents (Morrow, 1976). In the course of their development, children internalise the values held by parents. It follows that subsequent loss of control is detrimental to self respect. The term 'clean', in a symbolic sense, implies goodness, honesty and reliability, whereas being 'unclean' means the opposite (Kretschmer, 1978). Our concept of what is 'normal' does not include the collection of urine or faeces in a bag attached to the abdomen (Abrams, 1984). Kelly (1985) describes how his reaction to surgery was triggered by leakage from his appliance:

> 'For the rest of the day I felt utterly wretched, sad and overwhelmed by a sense of loss and failure. I was not upset by the loss of my bowel *per se* but rather by the loss of its function. My sense of failure came from viewing my body as having been wrecked by surgery.' (pp. 520–521)

The loss of self-esteem which may follow stoma surgery may be accompanied by fears of rejection and of being ostracised. For many patients being an ostomate can mean rejection by friends, the end of a sexual relationship or even marital breakdown (Morrison, 1981). The fear of an embarrassing accident with soiling or smell can be very great (Abrams, 1984). Kelly writes:

> 'What really alarmed me were the physiological consequences, especially the incontinence and the smell. These I believed would become the defining characteristics of my social identity and everything about me, my relationships, the way others viewed me, would be conditioned by these.' (p. 521)

However, the loss of control over elimination is just one aspect, for the ostomate endures loss on several counts: loss of autonomy on entering hospital, loss of a body part and sometimes loss of sexual function.

Studies with both animals and humans have shown that premature death may follow exposure to aversive outcomes when they cannot be controlled. Laboratory research has also shown that stress tolerance can be increased by the availability of distractors, information about the threatening event or by perceived control over aversive stimuli (Langer, 1983).

On entering hospital, patients relinquish control to their doctors and this, in itself, can be a source of stress, as situations that enforce passivity and dependency are known to be debilitating (Haan, 1982). The debilitation due to physiological imbalance is compounded by psychological upset. The patient is faced with an abrupt end to his usual life-style which has passed out of his control (Cohen and Lazarus, 1982). Whereas loss of control may give rise to anxiety, a chronic feeling of loss of control may give rise to passivity and giving up in the face of failure. This reaction, described as 'learned helplessness', is believed to be the root of reactive depression (Seligman, 1975). Therefore, it is not surprising that patients are often depressed following stoma surgery (Devlin et al, 1971; Kretschmer, 1978; MacDonald et al, 1982). An important question is, how do they adapt?

## Adaptation

The psychological implications of the surgical mutilation, which stoma surgery entails, have been likened to those of bereavement and it is suggested that a period of mourning and grief for the lost part of the body is to be expected (Barney, 1978). The length of time that it takes to adapt and to accept life with a stoma varies, but it is estimated that, like bereavement, it takes about one year. An uncomplicated recovery may make it easier, but in unfavourable cases the stoma may never be accepted. The transitional period between surgery and acceptance is emotionally painful (Meaney, 1985).

> 'Usually the first year after surgery can be classified as one of disability, with hospitalisation, experimentation, learning, fears of leaving home, relief at being alive, etc.' (Barney and Perlman, 1971, p. 115)

It would seem that if a patient has not resolved his 'hang ups' after 1 year he may well remain a psychological cripple for the rest of his life. Many patients are certainly left with a permanent sense of stigma (MacDonald et al, 1982).

The way in which patients react to surgery and adapt to their changed circumstances varies and patients may go through several stages in coming to terms with their stoma. For example, there may be an initial response of 'denial' before adjustment takes place (Devlin, 1984; Kelly, 1985). Such denial is manifest when a patient refuses, or is reluctant to look at his stoma, when a patient is loathe to assume responsibility for the care of his stoma, or when a patient, despite extensive preparation, denies being given information about the operation beforehand. Abrams (1984) maintains that much of this 'amnesia' is denial or selective hearing and that we should not be fooled by what appears to be understanding and acceptance. Devlin (1976) suggests that the development of a 'phantom rectum' may be associated with anal denial.

A different view of patient reactions is put forward by stoma care nurses who suggest that, initially, anxiety interferes with most peoples' ability to integrate and assimilate information and that, rather than avoiding informa-tion, there is a guarded confrontation as patients slowly and reluctantly face the reality of having to learn to care for the stoma (Bromley, 1980; Jackson, 1975).

Although the new ostomate is likely to be depressed, either overtly or covertly, the extent of this depression will vary according to the patient's personality. Thus the patient may be withdrawn and tearful, angry and aggressive or over-talkative and excessively cheerful.

Extreme reactions have also been described as patients attempt to come to terms with life with a stoma. The 'prisoner of the bathroom' is obsessed with cleanliness and develops elaborate and inflexible routines to care for his stoma, possibly as a substitute for control over bowel function (Morrow, 1976). The 'phobic social isolate' has also been described. This patient is overwhelmed by the constant fear of accidents and spillage. He avoids social rejection by restricting his interests and by withdrawing from emotional involvement (Morrow, 1976).

It would appear that adaptation to life with a stoma will depend on the length of time it takes to work through the grieving process. Kelly (1985) describes the stages outlined by Parkes (1972) which appeared to reflect his own experience:

- *realisation*—characterised by avoidance or denial of the loss followed by experiences of unreality or blunting;
- *alarm*—characterised by anxiety, restlessness, fear and insecurity;
- *searching*—characterised by acute episodic feelings of anxiety and panic and a preoccupation with the loss;
- *grief*—characterised by feelings of internal loss and multilation;
- *resolution*—characterised by efforts to construct a new social identity.

Having seen how patients adapt and approximately how long it takes to complete this process, two questions remain:

- What impact does a stoma care nurse make?
- What other factors make it easier, or harder to adapt to life with a stoma?


## Factors which may facilitate or hinder adaptation

### Age and sex

It is suggested that younger patients find it easier to adapt to life with a stoma. As patients who have an ileostomy are generally younger it is suggested that they tend to adapt better than patients who have a colostomy (Kretschmer, 1978; Devlin, 1984). Swaffield (1979) reports that younger people seem to demand more information about their condition and its management and are dissatisfied if they do not get it.

On the other hand, older people may have other disabilities such as poor sight, arthritis of the hands and mobility problems which can make caring for a stoma more difficult (Vowles, 1978). It may also be that older people cut down further on activities which they have already begun to reduce. They may curtail their sexual activity, for example (Swaffield, 1979).

Nevertheless, it appears that both age and gender may influence the degree to which ostomates become socially isolated. A number of British and American studies have shown that older people and women have the greatest difficulties with rehabilitation (Kretschmer, 1978). Devlin et al (1971) maintain that social isolation is greater for women in all age groups.


### Type of admission

In this framework for analysis, it is not the reason for the emergency surgery that is considered, but the implications of the sudden event for the eventual rehabilitation of the ostomate.

Abrams (1984) suggests that there is almost never too much time to prepare a patient and his family emotionally for a permanent stoma:

> 'In my experience the worst results, psychologically, have been with patients who have either received no preparation or were too sick to be prepared or who have been given inaccurate or dishonest information.' (Abrams, 1984, p. 39)

A considerable proportion of ostomates undergo emergency surgery. Devlin (1984) estimates that approximately 30% fall into this category and says that nursing and medical attitudes are crucial to long-term success for these cases. When a patient undergoes emergency surgery the time for preoperative preparation and teaching is either grossly reduced or non-existent. Thus, it would seem that many patients are left with a stoma without either understanding or, in some cases, even knowing beforehand of the possibility that this might happen. Therefore, it is not surprising that patients may subsequently feel that they have been assaulted, or be unable to accept a stoma that they never agreed to have in the first place (Morrison, 1978).

Clearly, it would seem that the obstacles to adaptation and rehabilitation are greater for those who undergo emergency surgery.

*Information*

Two issues are involved here. The first is the extent to which patients are prepared or given information and the second is the extent to which patients are satisfied with the information they are given. Moreover, ostomates may be given information of at least three kinds. The first relates to information about their disease and includes diagnosis and prognosis. The second type of information covers the reasons for stoma surgery, what it entails, the purpose of investigative tests and what to expect when recovering from surgery. The third kind of information relates to self-care and includes information about different types of appliance, how to obtain and dispose of appliances, care of the stoma and sources of help if problems should arise.

Janis and Rodin (1982) suggest that people seek causal attributes which may be erroneous if symptoms are unfamiliar and difficult to interpret. Thus, cancer patients may attribute their illness to some past experience. Such misattributions may lead to self-blame, but if they are counterbalanced by realistic information people are less likely to delay treatment and feel more adequate and less dependent (Abrams and Finesinger, 1953). On the other hand, Cohen and Lazarus (1982) state that, whereas some patients are insatiable in their search for information, others avoid it and prefer to place themselves in the hands of someone they can trust. Therefore, it would seem that the decision to tell or not to tell a patient his diagnosis and/or prognosis is less important than satisfying the patient's wishes with regard to information.

The perceived loss of control experienced by ostomates, which can lead to anxiety or passivity and giving up in the face of failure, has already been discussed. Janis and Rodin (1982) maintain that:

• preparatory information may function as a form of stress inoculation if it enables people to develop effective resources and coping mechanisms thus increasing their stress tolerance;
• the explanations that individuals receive for their illness and treatment profoundly affect their expectations of successful recovery and, possibly, the degree to which they take appropriate actions to contribute to their own improvement.

There is some evidence to support this view. Wilson-Barnett and Osborne (1983) review a representative selection of evaluative studies in patient teaching. Teaching, in this instance, refers to an interactive process wherein information is given systematically and levels of knowledge are checked, and, of the 29 studies reviewed, 23 appeared to show some benefits to patients. The authors suggest that anxiety is alleviated by reducing the areas of unknown experiences, fears and fantasies by providing a realistic account of what will happen and that instruction helps patients to know what is expected of them and how to do things which will improve their experiences and recovery. They can then behave in a useful way and feel less helpless and dependent.

It would seem that patient satisfaction with information may be associated positively with subsequent adaptation.

### Trade-off

It is suggested that patients with a long-standing debilitating disease such as ulcerative colitis, which has severely curtailed both work and leisure activities, will consider colectomy and ileostomy as a reasonable trade-off in exchange for health and the joys of living. This trade-off is easier for those who have been sicker for a longer period of time (Abrams, 1984). Ulcerative colitis gives rise to several disabling complications, such as fistulae, pseudopolyps, perforation and malabsorption. Surgery brings relief from these complications and from the pattern of remissions and exacerbations which characterise what has been termed a 'nerve-wracking' disease (Barney and Perlman, 1971). As some of these patients may come to surgery at their own request, the ileostomy may be regarded as a minor inconvenience after a life of misery (Irving, 1982).

The possibility of trade-off for cancer patients is less clear. Brady (1984) suggests that patients who have been relatively asymptomatic, but who are found to have cancer of the rectum for which surgery is required without delay, face a double blow. They have to cope with knowledge of the disease and with a stoma. For these patients, surgery is an abrupt and shocking procedure required to save life (Barney and Perlman, 1971). Druss et al (1969) suggest that these patients can be expected to feel worse than they did before surgery. On the other hand, their chief concern is the possibility of cure and it may be that in the immediate postoperative period they will be less concerned about the actual stoma (Donaldson, 1976). Although there may be some trade-off for these patients in the short-term, the evidence from a study of long-term survivors of surgery suggests that successful adaptation is rare (MacDonald et al, 1982).

### The temporary stoma

With regard to adaptation, the nature or reason for giving a patient a temporary, instead of a permanent, stoma may be less important than the implications of being told that a stoma is going to be temporary. Little is known about the incidence and outcome for patients with temporary stomas, although information from appliance manufacturers suggests that this operation is more commonly performed in the UK (Devlin, 1984). Data from one hospital show that almost one half of all colostomies were deemed 'temporary' but that almost one half of these were not closed because of inoperable disease. However, figures from Sweden showed that approximately three quarters of patients had their 'temporary' stomas closed. The time interval to closure varied between three weeks and three years (Nordstrom and Hulten, 1983).

From the patients' point of view the implications of being told that a stoma is 'temporary' may be considerable. Whereas the reversal of a temporary stoma may be seen as the 'finishing touch' by the surgeon, the patient may wait anxiously for the final step in returning him to normality (Kretschmer, 1978). It seems likely that, if patients anticipate a return to normal, a decision not to reverse the stoma could be quite devastating.

It has been suggested that the temporary ostomate may defer taking responsibility for the care of his stoma or even refuse to do so (Young, Wood and Watson, 1977). Temporary ostomates may also prefer to withdraw from social or emotional involvement until such time as the stoma is closed. Breckman (1980) says that many patients fear that, if they become too well, the doctors will not close their stoma. Young, Wood and Watson (1977) suggest that the temporary ostomate may become the lost soul who has limited access to the resources that are available to those with a permanent colostomy, and they point out that the sudden loss of control and change in body image are catastrophic events for people with either a permanent or a temporary stoma.

A further problem arises from the need to wear an appliance. As Devlin (1984) points out, a temporary (loop) colostomy is bulky, it needs support at stem level to ensure complete distal defunction and this makes it difficult to fit an appliance. The site of such stomas between the navel and the costal margins may add to this difficulty (Nordstrom and Hulten, 1983).

Therefore, it would seem that, in addition to the difficulties in fitting an appliance, being told that a stoma is temporary may have negative implications with regard to adaptation and acceptance by the patient if the surgeon subsequently decides that closure is inadvisable.

*Family support*

In a review of the literature on coping, Cohen and Lazarus (1982) state:

> 'There is growing evidence that ailing people do better in many ways if they can maintain and utilise social relationships. Social supports appear to enhance the possibilities for effective coping.' (p. 221)

None of the available social supports is more important than that of the patient's close family, especially his spouse or partner. To some extent the way in which we see ourselves is derived from the attitudes others have towards us. The change in body image and the feelings of shame or mutilation experienced by some ostomates render the support of a spouse or other close relative even more important than it had been previously. Kretschmer (1978) maintains that stoma surgery can have repercussions on the whole family who need to understand the implications of having a stoma so that they can give this support. Abrams (1984) points out that the idea of a stoma may be repulsive to both the patient and his family so that failure to work with them can be disastrous.

It appears that isolated patients, with no-one to depend on, are more at risk of becoming depressed and of cutting themselves off even more following surgery. It may also be the case that the widowed individual is already in a stigmatised social position which may be compounded by having a stoma and/or cancer (MacDonald and Anderson, 1984). Therefore, it is not surprising that the availability of a spouse is seen as the key to success or failure for the ostomate (Barney, 1978; Druss et al, 1969; Kretschmer, 1978; Prudden, 1971; Wilson, 1981).

## Readmissions/complications

A not inconsiderable proportion of patients may be readmitted for further surgery. The rate of complications such as parastomal hernia or prolapse is higher for loop colostomies than for end-sigmoid colostomies (Kretschmer, 1978; Chandler and Evans, 1978; Nordstrom and Hulten, 1983). Most of these complications occur during the early postoperative period. Chandler and Evans (1978) point out that loop colostomies prolapse 10 times more frequently than end colostomies. Surgery for initial obstruction appeared to be the predisposing factor. Thus, it would appear that emergency admissions for obstruction may be more likely to be given a temporary stoma and may also be more prone to complications.

## The stoma care nurse

A nurse specialist in stoma care is a nurse with special knowledge and expertise who has completed a recognised course in stoma care. Her task is to instruct and educate patients and staff in the principles and practice of stoma care and to ensure continuity of care for patients with all types of stoma. It is necessary to go into some detail regarding the role of the stoma care nurse as this is crucial to an understanding of the design of this study. The role components outlined below are those which have been described in books or papers written by stoma care nurses.

It is generally agreed that the stoma care nurse is primarily a clinician who aims to improve the quality of care given to patients who undergo stoma surgery by way of direct patient care, education/teaching and research.

The direct patient care aspect of the stoma care nurse's role is of prime interest in this patient-focused study. For those patients undergoing elective surgery this care begins in the outpatients department and continues after admission. The first task of the stoma care nurse is to establish rapport with the patient in preparation for the initial nursing assessment. The purpose of this assessment is to find out how the patient feels about his disease, body image and sexuality and to obtain information about his family and the stability of his relationships. Details of other conditions such as skin problems, arthritis, poor sight, allergies or obesity are also sought together with details of the patient's life style, work, leisure activities, home circumstances and amenities such as sanitation and refuse disposal.

The education and preparation of the patient begins as soon as possible and members of the patient's family are included in this if it is appropriate. The stoma care nurse works with the patient and his family to reinforce their own resources and to counter any fears, anxieties and cultural or personal taboos the patient may have and which interfere with his ability to integrate and assimilate information (Plant, 1976; Bromley, 1980). She explains the purpose of preoperative investigations and tests, the surgical procedure and what to expect immediately following surgery, for example, pain, nasogastric tubes, intravenous infusion, catheters and wound drainage (Meaney, 1985). Several visits to patients may be necessary before the nurse is satisfied that the patient has fully understood all the information given to him. She may use simple diagrams and booklets, to help clarify her explanation, which she can discuss with the patient.

Breckman (1977) cites four problem areas which need to be covered: acceptance of the disease, change of body image, how the patient thinks others seen him and psychosexual problems. More specifically Abrams (1984, p. 39) gives a list of questions which need to be worked through:

- Why do I need this stoma?
- Where will the stoma be sited?
- How does the stoma work?
- Do I have to follow a special diet?
- How do I take care of the stoma?
- Can I bathe, go swimming and so on?
- Will I have to wear special clothes?
- How is this going to affect my marriage and other personal relationships such as at work or at social events?
- Will everybody know that I have a stoma?
- Will I be able to have intercourse and have children?

One of the most important preoperative tasks is the siting of the stoma itself.

'An improperly placed stoma is a potential disaster that can severely hinder an ostomy patient's postoperative rehabilitation or even make it impossible for him to manage his stoma care.' (Lerner et al, 1980, p. 48)

Clearly many authors consider that this is an important component of the stoma care nurse's role, although some suggest that both the surgeon and stoma care nurse should be involved in discussing this with the patient (Breckman, 1979b; Sredl, 1980; Stockley, 1982).

The position for the stoma is marked after the patient is seen bending, sitting and standing, taking care to avoid the navel, belt line, scars, bony prominences, abdominal creases and bulges. The patient must be able to see the stoma easily and consideration must be given to a patient's occupation, physical pursuits and the need to wear other appliances before the site is chosen. A pouch may be placed on the chosen site as a final check before surgery (Stockley, 1982). When the patient is lying flat, as on the operating table, it can be difficult to see where the stoma should be placed (Reeves, 1984). Thus, the siting of the stoma is more of a problem for those admitted for emergency surgery.

Broadwell (1983) points out that, although the technical aspect of fitting a pouch is only a small part of the stoma care nurse's role, if this is not done properly it can severely impair good rehabilitation. Psychological problems are difficult to deal with when patients are troubled by leakage and sore skin (Beadle, 1981).

In the early postoperative period, the stoma care nurse makes daily visits to the patient to evaluate management of the stoma and to coordinate patient care in consultation with ward staff (Jackson, 1980). She observes and assesses the stoma with regard to size, shape, colour and oedema, and fits a transparent drainable bag which allows for observation and management of the large volume of efflux which often occurs in the early period following a colostomy or an ileostomy. The appliance is chosen to provide maximum protection of the peristomal area. This is particularly important for ileostomies and ileal conduits (Abrams, 1984).

Initially, the patient may be reluctant to look at his stoma but it is important that he accepts the responsibility of caring for it himself. Working with the ward sister and other nursing staff the stoma care nurse encourages the patient to participate in caring for his stoma as soon as he is sufficiently recovered from surgery. Patients should not be discharged before reaching an adequate level of self-care with minimal assistance (Abrams, 1984). Wherever possible the stoma care nurse encourages a close relative to be present during instruction to ensure that there will be someone capable of caring for the patient if he should become ill (Plant, 1976).

Before discharge the stoma care nurse may give the patient a choice of bag. This reinforces the idea that he can take responsibility for himself and care for his stoma (Breckman, 1977). The patient with a descending or sigmoid colostomy may prefer a closed bag but a drainable bag is more appropriate for a transverse colostomy or an ileostomy. Additionally, the patient may choose between a 1-piece bag which attaches directly to the skin or to a peristomal wafer, or a 2-piece appliance. Before discharge the stoma care nurse supplies the patient with a list containing details of the chosen appliance and any necessary accessories such as flanges, filters, belts, adhesive squares or tape, clips, clamps, deodorants, bag covers and, for the patient with a urinary stoma, tubing and night drainage system. The patient is given at least a three week supply of equipment and is given the following information:

- how to obtain further supplies;
- how to store his equipment;
- how to dispose of used appliances.

The patient is also told that the stoma may reduce in size after a few weeks and that a different size of appliance may be needed.

In addition to teaching the patient how to care for his stoma and giving information on how to obtain new supplies and dispose of used appliances, the stoma care nurse provides information or advice, as appropriate, on the following areas (Breckman, 1979b; Jackson, 1980):

- irrigation;
- diet;
- fluid intake;
- medication such as bulking agents, laxatives or contraception;
- ways of coping with problems arising from chemotherapy or radiotherapy;
- travel and holidays;
- employment;
- how to contact the stoma care nurse;
- how to contact the appropriate voluntary organisation;
- resources available in the community;
- pregnancy;
- sexual activity.

At any stage in the patient's progress the stoma care nurse may arrange for a visit from an ex-patient, usually a member of an ostomy association, who has a well-established stoma. Such a volunteer is chosen carefully and matched if possible for age, sex and type of stoma (Stockley, 1982).

Continuity of care may be crucial to the rehabilitation of ostomates who may need strong support and encouragement if they are to return to work and take up the social activities they enjoyed before becoming ill (Breckman, 1977; Saunders, 1976). The stoma care nurse assesses the home conditions of the patient and mobilises services and resources as necessary. She also works to increase the ostomate's self confidence and self-esteem and responds to problems which may arise within the family, coordinating and liaising with other agencies as appropriate. The stoma care nurse also runs an outpatient stoma clinic which patients may attend and provides a telephone service so that patients may obtain advice or help quickly when the need arises.

Some patients may develop postoperative complications such as prolapse, retraction or stenosis of the stoma, fistulae, herniation, urinary infections or fluid or electrolyte imbalance. Complications are more likely to occur in the first twelve months following surgery, and the stoma care nurse ensures that patients will recognise the signs and symptoms of conditions which require medical aid (Plant, 1976).

The stoma care nurse identifies and gives extra support to those patients who have specific problems such as arthritis or poor sight or those who are terminally ill. Ostomates who do not have these problems initially may develop them in later life when they may give rise to management problems. Continuing care should, therefore, continue as necessary for the rest of the ostomate's natural life (Plant, 1976).

According to Brady (1985) the stoma care nurse must never miss an opportunity to teach. This is especially important with regard to nurses on the ward as they have to care for the patient when she is elsewhere (Broadwell, 1983). Thus, the stoma care nurse instructs not only the patients and their relatives on the practical aspects of stoma care and appliances but she also teaches the nursing staff and educates nurses on the types of problems faced by patients, teaching them how to recognise and allay the fears and anxieties of individual patients.

In addition to these activities, the stoma care nurse works to ensure that her role is understood by all the people who may be involved in the care of ostomates, for example, general practitioners, chemists and patients' associations (Breckman, 1979b). She plans, organises and participates in training programmes, study days, seminars and conferences, in order to continually update her own knowledge. She then conveys all the relevant information to medical and nursing staff or other interested groups, and this can often be achieved by liaising with manufacturers (Saunders, 1976).

Research is the third component of the stoma care nurse's role which has been derived from the literature. In order to be able to evaluate her practice, the stoma care nurse maintains a comprehensive system of patient records. These enable quantification of the number of ostomates and of their needs. In addition to helping manufacturers to improve their products by participating in clinical trials (Breckman, 1979), stoma care nurses should evaluate the quality and the cost effectivenesss of the care that they give (Jackson, 1980).

In describing the future role of the stoma care nurse, Brady (1985) suggests that they will manage their own budgets and prove their cost-effectiveness within that budget, submitting reports to management with recommendations for improving the standard of nursing care.

There is, as yet, no direct evidence to support the view that patients who receive specialist nursing care adapt to life with a stoma better than those who do not. It seems likely, from the patients' point of view, that the stoma care nurse is seen as a valuable resource, providing information, reassurance, encouragement, a well-fitting appliance and continuity of care. Therefore, the stoma care nurse is regarded as a positive factor with regard to adaptation and rehabilitation.

## Discussion

So far, the discussion has hinged upon the possible single influence of patient attributes or events on eventual adaptation. On reflection it is apparent that some of these factors are related (Figure 1.1). For example, women tend to live longer than men and it is therefore probable that within any group of old people there are likely to be more widows than there are widowers. If, as alleged, having a spouse is the key to success or failure in adapting to life with a stoma, then it will be necessary to take marital status into account when looking at sex differences in adaptation.

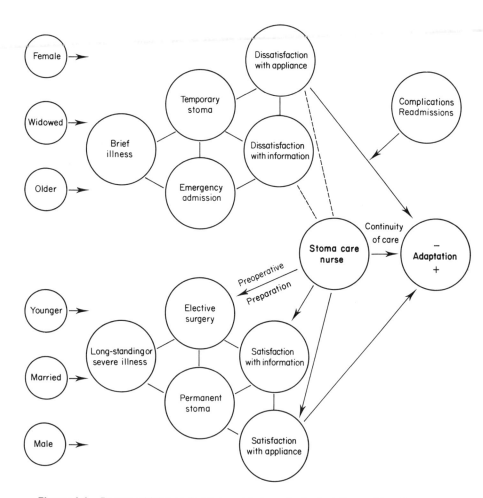

**Figure 1.1**   Factors which may facilitate or hinder patient adaptation to life with a stoma

Other anticipated relationships are indicated by the solid lines in Figure 1.1, although some of these other relationships are perhaps less obvious than the example just given. It seems probable that patients who have been ill for a long time are more likely to be admitted for elective surgery. It also seems likely that list cases will be better informed and will, in consequence, be more satisfied with the information that they are given than patients admitted for emergency surgery. For these patients the time for preoperative preparation is extremely limited and they may also be too ill to comprehend the information. To complicate matters even further, it would seem that there is also less time to prepare the families of these patients so that they can give the support which appears to be so important to the future welfare of the patient.

When these factors are considered, together with the notion of 'trade-off', those patients who are younger, married, have been ill for a longer period of time and are admitted for elective surgery would appear to be more likely to become reconciled to life with a stoma than an older patient who lacks the support of a spouse and who is admitted for emergency surgery.

However, the matter does not even rest there. It is alleged that some temporary ostomates may defer resumption of their previous life-style in anticipation of a return to normal. It would seem that this is another factor which must be taken into account. Moreover, it would appear that temporary transverse colostomies are more prone to complications, perhaps requiring readmission, and are less suited to the wearing of an appliance. These additional problems may make acceptance of the stoma even more difficult.

Into this rather complicated theoretical network, we must now introduce a further factor, the stoma care nurse, and consider the effects that she may have on the relationships described. These effects are indicated by the broken lines in Figure 1.1. Although the stoma care nurse may be unable to prepare patients for emergency surgery it may be that, by recognising those patients who will find it more difficult to adapt to life with a stoma, she may to some extent compensate for the additional disadvantages that have been described. For example, she may give more intensive counselling to older patients, especially those who are widowed. Similarly, she may concentrate more of her efforts into the postoperative care of those who have undergone emergency surgery. She may also counsel the 'temporary' ostomate with a view to achieving acceptance of the stoma as a safeguard for the strong possibility that the stoma may become permanent.

If the presence of a stoma care nurse does compensate those groups of patients who appear to be especially at a disadvantage then they may, in the long-term, fare little or no worse than other less disadvantaged patients. On the other hand, such patients may be expected to do less well when there is no stoma nurse to give this extra care. The possibility of the 'interaction effect' indicated by the broken lines in Figure 1.1 will be explored in later analysis.

## Summary

The factors which may influence the degree to which patients adapt to life with a stoma have been identified from the literature. The following hypotheses are derived:

- *age*—younger people may adapt more readily than those who are older;
- *sex*—men may adapt more readily than women;
- *type of admission*—those who undergo elective surgery may adapt more readily than those who are admitted for emergency surgery;
- *information*—patients who are satisfied with the information they are given may adapt more readily than those who are not;
- *length of illness*—patients who have been ill for a longer period of time before surgery may adapt more readily than those who have been ill for a shorter period of time;
- *permanence of stoma*—those who understand that their stoma is permanent may adapt more readily than those who understand that their stoma is temporary;
- *marital status*—patients who have the support of a spouse may adapt more readily than those who do not;
- *uncomplicated recovery*—patients whose recovery is relatively uncomplicated may adapt more readily than those who suffer complications/physical symptoms;
- *access to a stoma care nurse*—patients who have access to a stoma care nurse may adapt more readily than those who do not.

The description of the work of the stoma care nurse also suggests that patients in stoma nurse districts will be more satisfied with the information they have been given and will have greater knowledge of and be more independent in self care. They will have fewer appliance problems and will be more satisfied with their appliances. Family involvement will also be greater for these patients than for patients in other districts.

# 2

# The Design of the Study

## with Elaine Bielby

In 1982, a preliminary postal survey of all health districts in England and Wales was carried out to identify the number and function of clinical nurse specialists. Replies were received from 194 of the 202 districts (8 of these were refusals) which represented a response rate of 92%. The information received indicated that 60% of districts were employing clinical nurse specialists in stoma care. The majority of these specialists had responsibility for a specific patient group or caseload, and provided advice to patients throughout the district with the objective of ensuring continuity of care for patients following their discharge from hospital.

Preliminary information obtained from stoma care nurses suggested that, on average, between 10 and 15 new patients are referred to stoma care nurses each month. If interviews were carried out at approximately 10 weeks, some interviews would be gained with patients whose stomas were temporary and a period of 1 year after surgery would be appropriate for second interviews.

### The pilot study

Aims and objectives

The aims and objectives of the study were:

(1) to test the feasibility of the proposed sampling procedure for the main study;

(2) to estimate the required sample size for the main study, calculated on the basis of variance on the measures devised for use in the study;

(3) to devise interview schedules for use with:
- stoma patients;
- stoma care nurses;
- other members of the health care team;

(4) to devise and refine measures to assess:
- physical state in terms of frequency/severity of symptoms;

- social constraints;
- perceived quality of life.

(5) to develop and refine measures of patient satisfaction and problems with appliances. These were based on preliminary work carried out with the RCN Stoma Care Forum for the purpose of assessing new or refined stoma care products;

(6) to assess the suitability for use in the main study of an abbreviated interview schedule for the assessment of anxiety and depression. This measure has been used in a study of patients following mastectomy (Maguire et al, 1978).

## Method

Requests for permission to carry out the pilot study were made to 6 health districts situated in London and the home counties. Due to delay in receiving approval from the Ethics Committees of 2 districts, the pilot study was conducted in 4 districts only, 2 of which employed stoma care nurses. Surgeons were approached with requests for permission to interview patients and visits were made to each district to explain the sampling procedure.

## Sample

Each district was asked to supply a list of patients who had undergone stoma surgery between 8 and 12 weeks prior to data collection. Letters were then sent to 45 patients requesting their help and cooperation with the research and of these individuals the results were as follows:

- 30 patients agreed to participate and were interviewed;
- 1 patient agreed to participate but was not interviewed;
- 1 patient had been readmitted to hospital;
- 2 patients had had the stoma closed;
- 1 patient had died;
- 6 patients did not respond.

Thus, as a proportion of possible interviews, the response rate was 73%. One of the interviews, with the parent of a baby who had undergone stoma surgery, was subsequently excluded from analysis due to the large amount of missing data.

## Measures

The patient interview schedule was designed to yield the following information.

(1)  Demographic details:
   - age;
   - sex;
   - marital status;
   - education/employment;
   - duration of illness;
   - type of stoma.

(2)  Care received before and after discharge from hospital:
   - visits/preparation/information received in hospital and the source of this information;
   - home visits by staff and volunteers;
   - patient visits to clinics.

(3)  Appliances:
   - type of appliance used;
   - self-care ability and need for help;
   - problems with appliance;
   - comfort and satisfaction with appliance.

(4)  Physical problems encountered/resolved since stoma surgery, e.g. pain, nausea, bleeding, infections.

(5)  Dietary changes.

(6)  Difficulties in activities of daily living.

(7)  Changes in social activities.

(8)  Quality of life.

(9)  Open-ended questions designed to elicit information relating to the experience of stoma surgery.

**Table 2.1**  Pilot study sample: age, sex and type of stoma

|  |  | Districts with stoma nurses (n = 19) | Districts without stoma nurses (n = 10) |
|---|---|---|---|
| Age | Mean | 61.6 | 59.2 |
|  | Standard deviation | 14.7 | 17.3 |
| Sex | Male | 10 | 6 |
|  | Female | 9 | 4 |
| Type of stoma | Ileostomy | 2 | 2 |
|  | Colostomy | 15 | 3 |
|  | Urostomy | 1 | 5 |
|  | 2 stomas | 1 | 0 |

## Analysis and results

Analyses were undertaken on the unit microcomputer (Apple), using a statistical package devised by M Bland (St George's Hospital, London).

The characteristics of patients in the two types of district (with or without a stoma care nurse) are given in Table 2.1. It can be seen that the two groups were clearly disparate with regard to type of stoma and this precluded meaningful comparisons.

## Refinement of measures

### Self-care information scale

The items included in this scale were derived from the literature and from discussions with stoma care nurses. The scale comprised questions about information that should be given to patients before they are discharged from hospital, and each item was coded according to the source of the information received. The method worked well during the pilot study and showed promise as a measure suitable for inter-group comparisons. The list of items was therefore expanded to make it more comprehensive and items which were not applicable to all patient groups were excluded. The range of scores on the revised scale is 0–12 (items 33–44 in the revised schedule, appendix).

### Problems and satisfaction with appliance

(1) *Appliance problems scale (APS)* This scale consisted of five specific questions relating to problems with the appliance. The items were taken from an item bank developed in collaboration with the RCN Stoma Care Forum. Responses to these questions were on a 3-point scale. Two of the five items were not suitable for patients with urinary stomas and these were replaced by two other items. The range of scores on the revised schedule is 5 to 15. (Items 74–78 in the appendix.)

(2) *Satisfaction with appliance scale (SAS)* This scale consisted of three visual analogue scales relating to overall comfort, ease of fixing and satisfaction with appliance. It was found that these scales were easy to administer when the patient was shown an example. Following the pilot study a further scale, relating to confidence in the appliance, was also included. Scores on the overall scale range from 0–400. (Items 82–85 in the appendix).

### Physical symptoms scale (PSS)

In the pilot study, patients were required to respond to questions relating to the perceived severity of physical problems encountered and/or resolved following discharge from hospital e.g.:

*Q*. Have you had any problems with diarrhoea?
   Was this troublesome? (rated 1–5)
   Is this still troublesome? (rated 1–5)

Thus, two sets of scores were recorded for each patient. The first of these relates to the number and frequency of problems encountered since discharge from hospital (**PPSA**). The second relates to the number and frequency of problems experienced at the time of interview (**PPSB**).

It was found that the wording of these questions rendered them insensitive and patients were reluctant to admit to having problems. In the revised schedule these items were reworded, e.g.:

*Q*. Have you had any pain?
   How often did you have this? (rated 1–5)
   Do you still get this pain now? How often? (rated 1–5)

A number of additional symptoms were noted during the pilot study and these were added to the revised schedule. Provision was made for the addition of further unlisted symptoms in the revised schedule (items 92–148 in the appendix).

### Activities of daily living

Specific questions about activities of daily living appeared too insensitive to use as a measure of outcome. This was due, mainly, to the wide variation in age and the disparity in activities between males and females. In order to keep the interview to a reasonable length, it was decided that this measure should be omitted from the revised schedule. Instead, a more general question ('Is there anything that you used to enjoy doing that you feel you can't do now?') was substituted in the revised schedule.

### Social constraints scale

This measure consisted of a list of social activities. Patients were asked to respond on a 5-point scale with regard to how often they engaged in these activities both before surgery and at the time of interview. In order to control for individual differences in sociability an ipsative scoring scheme was devised whereby the sum of the differences in the two sets of scores is divided by the number of different social activities engaged in before surgery. A constant of 10 is then added to the resulting score. Essentially, this method uses an individual as his own control and embodies the assumption that, where a person had only one activity before surgery, this was as important to that person as four or five activities might be to someone else. Following the pilot study further social activities were added to the list and provision was made for additional activities to be added during interview (items 155–179 in the revised schedule).

*Quality of life*

This measure consisted of three visual analogue scales designed to assess activity level, enjoyment of life and happiness. The patient was asked to make comparisons with his activity level, enjoyment of life and happiness before surgery. The patient was shown examples of completed scales and was told that a mark in the centre of the line would signify no change (items 184–186 in the revised interview schedule).

*The present state examination (PSE)*

Psychological adjustment was assessed using the PSE (Wing et al, 1974) using diagnostic criteria for anxiety and depression described by Feighner et al (1972). Inter-rater reliability was calculated and weighted kappa coefficients of 0.92 (Hall, 1974) were obtained for assessment of major depressive disorder and for depressive neurosis. A copy of the interview schedule is included in the appendix.

*Test–retest reliability*

Following refinement of the measures a separate small scale study was carried out to assess the test–retest reliability of those measures retained or modified for use in the main study.

Ethical approval and surgeons' permission was obtained to interview patients who had had stoma surgery at one of the London teaching hospitals. Over a period of 18 months a sample of 20 patients consented to interview. Each person was interviewed 10 weeks after surgery and again 2 weeks later. One person who was blind was unable to complete the visual analogue scales. Pearson product moment correlation coefficients were calculated from the two sets of scores. These, together with the means and standard deviations, are given in Table 2.2.

**Table 2.2**  Test-retest reliability of measures used in the main study

|  | First interviews | | | Second interviews | | |
|---|---|---|---|---|---|---|
|  | n | m | s.d. | m | s.d. | Pearson *r* |
| Self-care information scale (SCIS) | 20 | 8.45 | 1.83 | 8.85 | 1.90 | 0.94 |
| Appliance problems scale (APS) | 20 | 7.25 | 1.81 | 7.40 | 1.80 | 0.74 |
| Satisfaction with appliance scale (SAS) | 19 | 307.10 | 57.80 | 305.50 | 59.20 | 0.80 |
| Physical symptoms scale A (PSS) | 20 | 14.60 | 5.96 | 13.40 | 6.13 | 0.78 |
| Physical symptoms scale B (PSS) | 20 | 9.65 | 4.49 | 8.45 | 4.14 | 0.57 |
| Social constraints scale (SCS) | 20 | 10.93 | 1.04 | 10.73 | 0.84 | 0.90 |
| Quality of life scale (QLS) | 19 | 131.70 | 50.49 | 141.6 | 53.70 | 0.70 |

At 10 weeks following surgery, patients are not usually fully recovered and some improvement may be expected for most patients in the interval between tests. This effect is apparent in the results given for the physical symptoms scale (B) which relates to symptoms experienced at the time of interview. The correlation of 0.57 obtained for this scale represents the reliability of the measure having accounted for both error and physical change. A similar attenuation may account for the somewhat lower correlation of 0.7 obtained for the quality of life scale which asks patients to assess their activity level, enjoyment and happiness relative to what it was before surgery.

## Conclusion

Following completion of the pilot study a meeting of the Scientific Advisory Group to the project was held to discuss the findings and methods for the main study. It was decided that in the main study:

- A 'link' person should be established in each district to supply patient lists.
- Patients under the age of 16 and those for whom the prognosis was very poor should be excluded from the main study.
- A stratified random sample of 24 health districts would be included in the main study. Twelve districts would be randomly selected from a list of all those districts in which stoma care nurses were employed and a further 12 districts would be randomly selected from the remainder.
- The patient sample would be proportionate to the size of health districts.
- Refinements to the measures described above precluded estimation of the required sample size from pilot study data. A preliminary target of 350 first phase interviews was set.
- First interviews with patients would be held at 10 weeks following surgery to enable some patients with temporary stomas to be included in the sample.
- Second interviews would take place one year later with sub-samples of patients from the two sets of districts. The sub-samples would be matched for age, sex and type of stoma.

It was also decided that the interview schedules were sufficiently comprehensive and of an appropriate length and that the measures which had been devised for inter-group comparisons should be more sensitive following the refinements described above.

### The main study

The initial design for the main study is shown in Table 2.3.

**Table 2.3**  Main study: target sample

|  | With stoma care nurses n | Without stoma care nurses n |
|---|---|---|
| Districts | 12 | 12 |
| Patients First interviews (10 weeks postoperative) | 176 | 176 |
| Second interviews (1 year later) | 50 | 50 |

## Method

A two stage sampling procedure was adopted wherein health districts would be randomly selected and patients would then be sampled from each district until the requisite number was obtained.

### The district sample

To allow for the possibility of refusals, approaches were made to 14 health districts which had been randomly selected from the list of those that employed stoma care nurses. One health district declined to take part, claiming staffing problems, and one was abandoned to leave 12 districts which were willing to participate in the study.

Envisaging a greater number of refusals from districts which did not employ stoma care nurses, approaches were made to 16 districts which had been randomly selected from the list. The request was refused by the surgical division in 2 districts, one district withdrew later and 4 districts were excluded as stoma care nurses were soon to be appointed. In 3 of these districts the decision to appoint a stoma care nurse was made known, after lengthy negotiations, when it was too late to make replacements. This left 9 districts which were willing to consider taking part in the study.

Initially, there was agreement to the research in principle. Following this, permission to proceed with the research was sought from ethics committees in all but one district. This particular district did not have such a committee and approval was given by the surgeons concerned. The time taken to obtain ethical approval varied from 1 month to 1 year, and there were similar delays in obtaining permission from the surgeons. The final response rate from the 114 surgeons approached was 90.4%.

After consent had been received from all the relevant individuals, including stoma care nurses and other nursing staff, a member of the research team visited each district to explain the sampling procedure, outline the information which would be required and to establish a 'link' person for that district. In the districts that employed stoma care nurses, the stoma care nurse usually acted as the link person. The link person in other districts was usually a ward sister or nursing officer.

## The patient sample

The sample size for each of the two sets of health districts was calculated proportionate to the size of the population of each district. The link person in each district was asked to provide lists of patients each month until the requisite sample was obtained. The information requested included:

- the name, address and, where possible, the phone number of each patient;
- the name of the consultant;
- the prognosis for each patient;
- the type of stoma (colostomy, ileostomy or urostomy);
- the date of surgery.

### Approach to patients

Letters were sent to the link person in each district stipulating which patients were to be approached from the list provided. Patients under the age of 16 years, those for whom the prognosis was very poor and those patients of surgeons who had refused to cooperate were excluded from the study.

Letters were sent to each of the remaining patients inviting them to participate in the study. The purpose of the research was explained and confidentiality was assured. A card was enclosed in each letter, together with a stamped addressed envelope. The card enabled patients to choose between the following responses:

- I agree to participate in the study.
- I do not wish to participate in the study.
- I am too ill to take part in the study.
- My stoma has been reversed.

Patients were asked to sign the card and to give a telephone number at which they could be contacted. They were also given a direct-line telephone number so that they could talk to a member of the research team and reverse the charges. Follow-up letters were sent to those patients who did not reply within two weeks.

Members of the research team established the protocol to be followed in the interviews. Pilot study taped interviews were examined and interview technique was practised using role play.

The patients who had agreed to take part were then contacted and appointments were made for a member of the research team to visit them at home. As far as possible patients were interviewed at 10 weeks following surgery. In some cases illness, convalescence, readmission or late lists meant that interviews were not carried out at exactly 10 weeks after surgery. Three patients were interviewed in hospital.

Before starting the interview, the purpose of the study was explained to patients again, and confidentiality was assured. In addition, patients were told that they could discontinue the interview at any time if they so wished, and they were asked if they would mind if some of their answers were tape-recorded. Each patient was allotted a code, so that names were not included on either the interview schedule or tapes. On completion of the interviews, patients were asked if they would agree to consider a further interview approximately 1 year later.

The first phase of interviews began in October 1983. Regular lists of patients were received from districts with stoma care nurses in post and few reminders were necessary. In the remaining 9 districts it proved more difficult to obtain the lists which were less regularly received. Occasionally, the link person moved and the task was given to someone else. The information received was not always complete and this also created problems. One district withdrew from the study after the first list when only one patient had been interviewed. In this particular district the permission of the surgeons concerned had been sought on our behalf by nursing staff and it was reported that they had second thoughts about providing lists of patients.

The second phase of interviews was due to start in October 1984, but because the sample from non stoma care nurse districts was incomplete it was impossible to match patients from the two samples. The number of ileostomates or urostomates was rather small and it was felt that all these patients should be reinterviewed. It was also felt that all those patients who understood that their stoma was temporary but who still had their stoma after 1 year should be reinterviewed. In January 1985, taking these factors into consideration it was decided to reinterview all survivors who had not had their stomas reversed. In April 1985, although the target sample for non stoma nurse districts was still incomplete, the list was closed. Altogether, approaches for the initial interviews had been made to 509 patients of which 25 had died, 34 replied that they were too ill, 34 had had their stomas reversed, 6 did not have a stoma and 22 patients had had surgery more than 13 weeks previously and were excluded. This left a possible sample of 388 patients of which 56 refused to participate and 68 did not respond. The remaining 264 patients were interviewed. Eighty-eight of these patients were in non stoma nurse districts and 176 were in stoma nurse districts. The response rate, calculated from the possible sample, was 68%.

After one year, 71 patients, of the 264 patients interviewed in the first phase, had had their stoma reversed, 10 were too ill to be interviewed and 42 patients

**Table 2.4**  The patient sample: required and obtained (calculated proportionate to size of population)

| | Districts with stoma nurses | | | | Districts without stoma nurses | | |
|---|---|---|---|---|---|---|---|
| | First interviews | | Second interviews | | First interviews | | Second interviews |
| District | Required | Obtained | Obtained | District | Required | Obtained | Obtained |
| 1 | 24 | 24 | 10 | 1 | 16 | 1 | 1 |
| 2 | 9 | 9 | 4 | 2 | 21 | 14 | 6 |
| 3 | 13 | 13 | 8 | 3 | 25 | 4 | 4 |
| 4 | 20 | 20 | 10 | 4 | 15 | 9 | 4 |
| 5 | 13 | 13 | 5 | 5 | 36 | 17 | 8 |
| 6 | 24 | 24 | 12 | 6 | 23 | 14 | 9 |
| 7 | 7 | 7 | 4 | 7 | 13 | 10 | 5 |
| 8 | 11 | 11 | 3 | 8 | 17 | 13 | 4 |
| 9 | 6 | 6 | 2 | 9 | 10 | 6 | 2 |
| 10 | 16 | 16 | 8 | | | | |
| 11 | 23 | 23 | 8 | | | | |
| 12 | 10 | 10 | 4 | | | | |
| Total | 176 | 176 | 78 | | 176 | 88* | 43* |

* One patient with 2 stomas was subsequently omitted from analysis

had died. This left a possible sample of 141 patients of which 3 refused to be interviewed and 4 did not respond. In the second phase, 121 patients were interviewed and of these 42 were in non stoma nurse districts. The late decision to reinterview all patients, together with staffing problems, meant that it was too late to contact 13 of the patients. The response rate for second interviews calculated from the possible sample of 141 patients was therefore 85.6%. The distribution of the patient sample for the districts included in the study is given in Table 2.4. It should be noted that one patient was found to have both a bowel stoma and a urinary stoma and was therefore excluded from analysis. A summary of the remaining sample, by type of stoma and type of district is given in Table 2.5.

### Interviews with staff

On completion of the patient interviews requests for interviews were made to the following individuals:

- 1 stoma care nurse in each of the stoma nurse districts;
- 1 surgeon in each district, randomly selected from the list;
- the Director of Nursing Services (Acute) or the equivalent;
- the Director of Nursing Services (Community) or the equivalent;
- 1 ward sister in each district.

**Table 2.5**  Number of patients who were reinterviewed, had their stomas reversed, were too ill, did not respond, or refused, by type of stoma

| | 10 week interview | Stoma reversed | Too ill | Died | Refused | No response | Not contacted | Reinterviewed | |
|---|---|---|---|---|---|---|---|---|---|
| | n | n | n | n | n | n | n | n | % |
| *Permanent colostomy* | | | | | | | | | |
| Stoma nurse | | | | | | | | | |
| Districts | 69 | 1 | 4 | 12 | 0 | 0 | 11 | 41 | 59.4 |
| Non stoma nurse | | | | | | | | | |
| Districts | 41 | 0 | 4 | 10 | 2 | 1 | 0 | 24 | 58.5 |
| All | 110 | 1 | 8 | 22 | 2 | 1 | 11 | 65 | 59.1 |
| *Temporary colostomy* | | | | | | | | | |
| Stoma nurse | | | | | | | | | |
| Districts | 73 | 48 | 0 | 7 | 1 | 3 | 0 | 14 | 19.2 |
| Non stoma nurse | | | | | | | | | |
| Districts | 32 | 20 | 1 | 5 | 0 | 0 | 0 | 6 | 18.8 |
| All | 105 | 68 | 1 | 12 | 1 | 3 | 0 | 20 | 19.0 |
| *Ileostomy* | | | | | | | | | |
| Stoma nurse | | | | | | | | | |
| Districts | 17 | 3 | 0 | 2 | 0 | 1 | 0 | 11 | 64.7 |
| Non stoma nurse | | | | | | | | | |
| Districts | 11 | 0 | 1 | 1 | 0 | 0 | 0 | 9 | 81.8 |
| All | 28 | 3 | 1 | 3 | 0 | 1 | 0 | 20 | 71.4 |
| *Urostomy* | | | | | | | | | |
| Stoma nurse | | | | | | | | | |
| Districts | 17 | 0 | 0 | 5 | 0 | 0 | 0 | 12 | |
| Non stoma nurse | | | | | | | | | |
| Districts | 3 | 0 | 0 | 0 | 0 | 0 | 0 | 3 | |
| All | 20 | 0 | 0 | 5 | 0 | 0 | 0 | 15 | 75.0 |
| *All stomas* | 263 | 72 | 10 | 42 | 3 | 5 | 11 | 120 | 45.6 |

The interviews with surgeons were designed to elicit information relating to policy issues such as the siting of stomas and giving information to patients, the appointment of stoma care nurses and the factors which might influence this. Questions were also included to ascertain attitudes towards increasing specialisation in nursing with special reference to stoma care nurses.

Interviews with directors of nursing services were also designed to clarify district policy with regard to the appointment of nurse specialists, the factors influencing such appointments and the attitudes of other staff to stoma care nurses and other nurse specialists.

Structured interview schedules were devised for use with ward sisters and stoma care nurses. These schedules were devised to provide the following information:

- length of time in post;
- training;
- case load and policy with regard to home visits;
- the care and information given to stoma patients;

- teaching activities;
- consultation by other staff;
- participation in research;
- publications.

Interviews were held with one stoma care nurse in each of the districts in which they were employed and with one ward sister or charge nurse in each district. Interviews were also held with directors of nursing services in all the districts included in the study. Interviews were obtained with 5 general surgeons in non stoma nurse districts and with 6 general surgeons and 2 urological surgeons in stoma nurse districts. These interviews were completed in November 1986.

### Analysis

Data were analysed on the University of London Amdahl computer using the Statistical Package for the Social Sciences version X.

Analysis of covariance was used to assess patient outcome with regard to the appliance problems scale, the appliance satisfaction scale, the social constraints scale and the quality of life scale. This method of analysis is particularly suited to a research design when it is not possible to randomly assign patients to groups. In this study, it is used to control for prior differences between subjects.

In addition to assumptions about normality and homogeneity of variance, analysis of covariance requires the assumptions of linearity, reliability of covariates and homogeneity of regression (Tabachnick and Fidell, 1983). Tests of these assumptions were made before analysis, and square root transformations were performed on scores on the physical symptoms scale and the measure of psychological adjustment which was also standardised.

The classic experimental approach (least squares) was used to take account of the differing sample size for the two sets of districts. In this approach covariates are assessed simultaneously first. Main effects are assessed after adjusting for covariates and other main effects. Interaction effects are examined last and are adjusted for covariates, main effects and lower level interaction effects.

### Summary

(1) A preliminary postal survey of all health districts in England and Wales revealed that 60% of health districts employed stoma care nurses.

(2) A pilot study was carried out in 4 health districts and measures were devised and refined to assess:

- self-care information;
- appliance problems;
- satisfaction with appliance;
- extent and severity of physical symptoms;
- social constraints;
- quality of life.

(3)  A small study was carried out to assess the test–retest reliability of the above measures. Inter-rater reliability was also established for a measure of psychological adjustment.

(4)  Twelve health districts which employed stoma care nurse were randomly selected and they agreed to take part in the study. From these districts, 176 patients were interviewed at 10 weeks following surgery and 78 patients were reinterviewed 1 year later.

(5)  Nine randomly selected health districts which did not employ stoma care nurses agreed to take part in the study and, of these, 1 later withdrew. Eighty-eight patients were interviewed from these districts at 10 weeks following surgery and 43 were reinterviewed 1 year later. One patient with 2 stomas was later excluded.

(6)  Based on the possible sample of patients the response rate was 68% for first interviews and 86% for the second interviews.

(7)  Interviews were obtained with 1 stoma care nurse from each of the 12 relevant districts. Interviews were also held with directors of nursing services and 1 ward sister in each participating district and with 13 surgeons who were randomly selected from participating districts.

# 3

# Patient Profile and Onset of Illness

'The doctor frowned and shook his head,
We'll have to operate, he said,
Within a month they'd done just that
And left me stitched up like a sack.'

### The patients

The target sample of patients from districts without stoma care nurses was not achieved (as described in the last chapter). To what extent, therefore, is the achieved sample representative?

We can approach this question in two ways. First of all we can calculate the average number of patients to each surgeon for the two sets of districts. For stoma nurse districts this was 2.51. The average for non stoma nurse districts was only slightly higher at 2.67.

More important, however, is the degree to which the sample obtained is representative of the population of stoma patients. The percentage distribution of the sample by type of stoma, together with the percentage distribution of types of stoma for the population is shown in Table 3.1. These figures were derived from industry sponsored market research and were presented at a seminar entitled 'The Future Role of Stoma Care' held in Copenhagen (Stringer, 1985).

It can be seen that the percentages shown are almost identical. On the basis of the above considerations it is reasonable to make the following conclusions:

- that the sample of patients included in this study is representative of the population of new ostomates;
- that the data from districts with and without stoma care nurses may be combined for analysis.

The percentage distribution of the sample by type of stoma for districts with and without stoma care nurses is given in Table 3.2. It can be seen that there are fewer urostomates from the non stoma nurse districts. However, taken as a

A Stoma is for Life

**Table 3.1** Percentage distribution of types of stoma within the population and within the sample

| Type of stoma | Market Research[1] New patients per year | | The sample | |
|---|---|---|---|---|
| | n | % | n | % |
| Permanent colostomy | 7 500 | 40.7 | 110 | 41.8 |
| Temporary colostomy | 7 500 | 40.7 | 105 | 39.9 |
| Ileostomy | 2 000 | 10.8 | 28 | 10.6 |
| Urostomy | 1 450 | 7.9 | 20 | 7.6 |
| Total | 18 450 | 100.1* | 263 | 99.9 |

[1] Stringer, 1985
* Due to 'rounding off' figures in this and subsequent tables figures do not always total exactly 100%

**Table 3.2** The distribution of ostomates by type of stoma for districts with and districts without stoma care nurses

| Type of stoma | Stoma care nurse districts | | Non stoma care nurse districts | |
|---|---|---|---|---|
| | n | % | n | % |
| Permanent colostomy | 69 | 39.2 | 41 | 47.1 |
| Temporary colostomy | 73 | 41.5 | 32 | 36.8 |
| Ileostomy | 17 | 9.7 | 11 | 12.6 |
| Urostomy | 17 | 9.7 | 3 | 3.5 |
| Total | 176 | 100.1 | 87 | 100.0 |

$\chi^2 = 4.58$, 3 d.f., n.s.

**Table 3.3** Age: means and standard deviations, by type of stoma and type of district

| Type of stoma | Stoma care nurse districts | | | Non stoma care nurse districts | | | All | | |
|---|---|---|---|---|---|---|---|---|---|
| | n | m | s.d | n | m | s.d. | n | m | s.d. |
| Permanent colostomy | 69 | 63.5 | 10.8 | 41 | 65.9 | 10.1 | 110 | 64.3 | 10.6 |
| Temporary colostomy | 73 | 61.3 | 13.8 | 32 | 63.9 | 12.2 | 105 | 62.1 | 13.4 |
| Ileostomy | 17 | 42.5 | 18.5 | 11 | 52.9 | 14.1 | 28 | 46.6 | 17.4 |
| Urostomy | 17 | 60.2 | 13.5 | 3 | 54.7 | 18.2 | 20 | 59.4 | 13.8 |
| Total | 176 | 60.2* | 14.4 | 87 | 63.4* | 12.6 | 263 | 61.3 | |

* t = 1.3, n.s.

whole, differences in the distribution of types of stoma between the two sets of districts are not statistically significant.

## Age

The mean (average) age of patients for each set of districts is shown, by type of stoma, in Table 3.3. The figures reveal an overall difference of 3 years between the two subsamples, with a greater difference in mean age for ileostomates and patients with urinary stomas. Taken overall, the difference between the mean age of patients from the two sets of districts is not statistically significant.

## Sex and marital status

The two subsamples of patients were not dissimilar with regard to the distribution of sex and marital status (Table 3.4). It was found that 55% of patients in stoma nurse districts were male compared to 52% in the other districts. In stoma nurse districts 69% of the patients were married compared with 68% in the other districts.

The main differences between the two subsamples seemed to be in relation to the number of patients with urinary stomas, their average age and the average age of ileostomates. As the number of urostomates is rather small and unevenly distributed between the two sets of districts, comparisons between stoma nurse districts and non stoma nurse districts will need to take account

**Table 3.4**  The sample: sex and marital status, by type of district

| Type of district | Marital status | Sex | | All |
| --- | --- | --- | --- | --- |
| | | Male % | Female % | % |
| | | n = 97 | n = 79 | n = 176 |
| With stoma care nurses | Single | 13.4 | 11.4 | 12.5 |
| | Married | 80.4 | 54.4 | 68.8 |
| | Widowed/divorced | 6.2 | 34.2 | 18.7 |
| | *Total* | 100.0 | 100.0 | 100.0 |
| | | n = 45 | n = 42 | n = 87 |
| No stoma care nurses | Single | 13.3 | 7.1 | 10.3 |
| | Married | 80.0 | 54.8 | 67.8 |
| | Widowed/divorced | 6.7 | 38.1 | 21.8 |
| | *Total* | 100.0 | 100.0 | 99.9 |

of this. As explained in the last chapter, the use of analysis of covariance to examine differences in patient outcome between the two sets of districts will enable control for intervening variables such as age or type of stoma.

## Events leading up to surgery

Fuller (1984) states:

'Carcinoma of the large bowel is the second commonest epithelial carcinoma in Britain. It is also the second commonest cause of death from cancer, despite the fact that there is ample evidence that early diagnosis improves prognosis.' (p. 825)

It would seem that the problem lies in achieving early diagnosis. According to Northover (1984), the prognosis in colorectal cancer has not changed for decades. At the stage that they are referred to the surgeon, half of the patients are beyond medical treatment and only one quarter will live for 5 years. The two most obvious reasons for delay are as follows:

- the patient neglects his symptoms and does not consult his physician;
- the general practitioner does not examine the patient or refer him for further investigation.

Both of these reasons are apparent from patient responses when they were interviewed and asked whether they had felt really ill before surgery and, if so, for how long. This particular question served as a trigger leading to a detailed account of the course of their illness including visits to their doctor and referral. The information presented in Table 3.5 indicates the length of time that patients, with different types of stoma, had felt really ill before being admitted to hospital. It is apparent that the pattern of illness differs for patients with different types of stoma; a greater proportion of ileostomates had been ill for a longer period of time. This information is of particular interest with regard to the notion of 'trade off' which will be explored in later analysis. It can also be seen that patients who had had abdominoperineal

**Table 3.5**  The length of time that patients felt really ill before surgery (and number of patients in each category), by type of stoma

| Type of stoma | | Number of weeks that patients felt really ill | | | | | All |
|---|---|---|---|---|---|---|---|
| | n | 0 % | 1–4 % | 5–13 % | 14–25 % | More than 26 % | % |
| Permanent colostomy | 110 | 51.8 | 11.0 | 14.5 | 10.9 | 11.8 | 100.0 |
| Temporary colostomy | 105 | 58.1 | 23.8 | 9.5 | 1.9 | 6.7 | 100.0 |
| Ileostomy | 28 | 28.6 (8) | 14.3 (3) | 25.0 (7) | 3.6 (1) | 28.6 (8) | 100.1 |
| Urostomy | 20 | 75.0 (15) | 5.0 (1) | 10.0 (2) | – | 10.0 (2) | 100.0 |

excision of rectum had a more extended pattern of illness than those who subsequently received a temporary colostomy. However, analysis of taped anecdotal data revealed that, although many patients had not felt really ill, they may have had some symptoms or they may have felt 'off colour' for varying lengths of time before surgery.

## Symptoms

The percentage of patients reporting different symptoms is shown, by type of stoma, in Table 3.6. It should be noted that these percentages are based on patient recall and it is likely that they underestimate the actual occurrence of symptoms. These symptoms also illustrate a different pattern for patients with different types of stoma. For example, the most frequently reported symptoms for those patients who subsequently received a permanent colostomy were pain, bleeding, diarrhoea and constipation, in that order. The frequency of reported pain and diarrhoea is almost identical for temporary colostomates, but bleeding was much less common and vomiting and obstruction were more commonly reported.

## Emergency admissions

We have seen that temporary colostomates tended to have felt ill for a shorter period of time and that they more frequently reported obstruction and vomiting. Therefore, it is not surprising that a greater proportion of these patients were admitted for emergency surgery. As this is an important variable

**Table 3.6**  Percentage of patients reporting different symptoms prior to surgery, by type of stoma

| Symptom | Permanent colostomy (n = 110) % | Temporary colostomy (n = 105) % | Ileostomy (n = 28) % | Urostomy (n = 20) % |
|---|---|---|---|---|
| Bleeding | 43.1 | 18.1 | 35.7 | 52.6 |
| Pain | 50.5 | 51.4 | 42.9 | 21.1 |
| Diarrhoea | 30.3 | 29.5 | 42.9 | 21.1 |
| Constipation | 18.3 | 16.2 | 7.1 | – |
| Obstruction | 10.1 | 19.0 | – | 5.3 |
| Vomiting | 0.9 | 13.3 | 17.9 | 5.3 |
| Frequency | 4.6 | – | – | 10.5 |
| Dysuria | 6.4 | 2.9 | – | 36.8 |
| Trauma | 0.9 | 2.9 | – | – |
| Other | 29.4 | 37.1 | 50.0 | 31.6 |

**Table 3.7**   Percentage of patients admitted for emergency surgery, by type of stoma and type of district

| Type of stoma | Stoma care nurse districts | | | Non stoma care nurse districts | | | All | | |
|---|---|---|---|---|---|---|---|---|---|
| | Emergency n | % | Elective % | Emergency n | % | Elective % | Emergency n | % | Elective % |
| Permanent colostomy | 69 | 11.6 | 88.4 | 41 | 9.8 | 90.2 | 110 | 10.9 | 89.1 |
| Temporary colostomy | 73 | 43.8 | 56.2 | 32 | 53.1 | 46.9 | 105 | 46.7 | 53.3 |
| Ileostomy | 17 | 5.9 | 94.1 | 11 | 18.2 | 81.8 | 28 | 10.7 | 89.3 |
| All bowel stomas | 159 | 25.8 | 74.2 | 85 | 28.2 | 71.8 | 244 | 26.6 | 73.4 |

with regard to later analysis, the number of patients admitted in this way is given for stoma nurse districts and non stoma nurse districts in Table 3.7.

## Discussion

It is already known that a greater proportion of patients who receive temporary stomas are admitted as emergencies. It might, therefore, be argued that these data are of academic interest. They are included as they demonstrate the gradual onset of illness for a considerable proportion of the sample.

Patients reported delay in seeing their doctor for a variety of reasons, including holidays, sick relatives or weddings. Often no reason for the delay was given. Others recounted seeing their physician on several occasions before being referred for further investigation. Two patients reported demanding a referral, one changed his GP and one was referred following the death of his doctor.

Northover (1984) describes an average delay of 6 months between the patient's first visit to his GP and the appropriate treatment in hospital. Hutchinson and Weston (1984) maintain that any patient over the age of 40 with a history of rectal bleeding or a change in bowel habit requires urgent investigation to exclude a colorectal cancer, and Brown (1984) suggests that sigmoidoscopy is an essential part of the routine investigation of such patients.

More than 15 years ago Devlin et al (1971), reporting a study of patients with anorectal cancer, commented that, although most patients were uncritical of their treatment, a few wondered why they had been treated at home for minor anorectal lesions for so long before being referred. It would seem that little has changed.

How can such delay be minimised in the future? Aldridge and Sim (1986) suggest that the only prospect of cure in colorectal cancer lies in its early diagnosis. Yet it would seem that the value of screening of symptom-free patients by testing for faecal occult blood is somewhat equivocal. Studies have shown a low diagnostic yield and compliance with screening may not be very high (Nichols et al, 1986).

A different approach was adopted by Chisholm et al (1985) who devised and refined a questionnaire for use in screening which they concluded could reliably elicit symptoms of gastrointestinal disease consistent with the ability of a clinician. Such a simple method has great appeal when, clearly, there is a need for earlier detection and referral. If this is to be achieved there is a need for patient education and for screening. Could this be undertaken by nurses?

## Summary

The following conclusions can be made.

(1) The distribution of the sample with regard to types of stoma closely resembles the distribution of types of stoma within the population of new ostomates (based on market research).

(2) The distribution of types of stoma between districts with stoma care nurses and those without differs slightly but the difference is not statistically significant.

(3) The mean age of the whole sample was 61 years with patients in stoma nurse districts being 3 years younger on average. The difference is not statistically significant.

(4) The distribution of sex and marital status is very similar for the two sets of districts.

(5) Emergency surgery had been performed on 27% of patients with bowel stomas. Almost one half of these understood that their stoma was temporary.

# 4

# Information Given
# to Patients:
# Their Recollections

'The nurses were as good as gold,
But the truth they seldom told;
The doctors were a bit aloof,
You really must not know the truth.'

In the first chapter three types of patient information were described. The first
of these was related to diagnosis and the reasons for stoma surgery, the second
to preoperative preparation and the third to postoperative self-care and
management of appliances. Each of these will now be considered and then
discussed in the light of patient satisfaction.

### Patients' recollections of their diagnoses

As background information to this section, a list of official diagnoses is given
in Table 4.1 with the appropriate percentages. The analyses described below
are based on patients' answers to two questions:

- Why did you have the operation?
- What did they tell you about the operation?

A very varied set of responses was revealed on analysis of the transcripts of
interviews given at approximately 10 weeks after surgery. These are shown in
Table 4.2. It can be seen that, whereas some patients could recall their actual
diagnoses, the responses of others were limited to lay explanations of the
surgical procedure. It is also evident that a considerable proportion of patients
(13.3%) either could not remember being given a diagnosis or said that they
had not been told.

It is interesting to compare what patients remembered about their
diagnoses to the official list given in Table 4.1. For example, it would appear

**Table 4.1**   Patient diagnosis (and number of patients), by type of stoma

| Diagnosis | Permanent colostomy (n = 110) % | Temporary colostomy (n = 105) % | Ileostomy (n = 28) % | Urostomy (n = 20) % |
|---|---|---|---|---|
| Carcinoma | 86.4 | 47.6 | 17.9 (5) | 80.0 (16) |
| Diverticular disease | 0.9 | 21.9 | 3.6 (1) | 0.0 |
| Ulcerative colitis | 0.0 | 0.9 | 35.7 (10) | 0.0 |
| Crohn's disease | 0.9 | 0.9 | 17.9 (5) | 0.0 |
| Trauma | 0.0 | 3.8 | 0.0 | 0.0 |
| Vascular disease | 0.0 | 2.9 | 0.0 | 0.0 |
| Abscess | 0.0 | 2.9 | 0.0 | 0.0 |
| Fistula | 0.0 | 1.9 | 0.0 | 0.0 |
| Fibrotic/inflammatory mass | 0.0 | 1.9 | 0.0 | 0.0 |
| Chronic constipation | 0.9 | 0.0 | 7.1 (2) | 0.0 |
| Rectal fissure | 0.0 | 0.9 | 0.0 | 0.0 |
| Perforated bowel | 0.0 | 0.9 | 0.0 | 0.0 |
| Faecal incontinence | 0.9 | 0.0 | 0.0 | 0.0 |
| Ovarian tumour | 0.0 | 0.9 | 0.0 | 0.0 |
| Polyposis | 0.9 | 0.0 | 3.6 (1) | 0.0 |
| Intussusception | 0.0 | 0.9 | 0.0 | 0.0 |
| Neurogenic bladder | 0.0 | 0.0 | 0.0 | 10.0 (2) |
| Spina bifida | 0.0 | 0.0 | 0.0 | 5.0 (1) |
| Unknown | 9.1 | 11.4 | 14.3 (4) | 5.0 (1) |
| *Total* | 100.0 | 99.7 | 100.1 | 100.0 |

Information was not obtained for 27 patients (10.3% of the whole sample)

**Table 4.2**   Patient recollections of diagnosis/reason for surgery

| Patient recollections | n | % | Patient recollections | n | % |
|---|---|---|---|---|---|
| Cancer | 53 | 20.2 | Fissure | 1 | 0.4 |
| Growth/tumour | 40 | 15.2 | Cyst | 1 | 0.4 |
| Ulcer | 18 | 6.8 | Sore | 1 | 0.4 |
| Blockage | 17 | 6.5 | Blood clot bowel artery | 1 | 0.4 |
| Ulcerative colitis | 14 | 5.3 | Benign cancer | 1 | 0.4 |
| Abscess | 11 | 4.2 | Inflamed bowel | 1 | 0.4 |
| Remove part of bowel | 10 | 3.8 | Bladder infection | 1 | 0.4 |
| Diverticulitis | 10 | 3.8 | Retention | 1 | 0.4 |
| Crohn's disease | 6 | 2.3 | Kidney disease | 1 | 0.4 |
| Perforation | 5 | 1.9 | Tear in the bowel | 1 | 0.4 |
| Polyps | 4 | 1.5 | 2/3 more bowel than most | 1 | 0.4 |
| Trauma | 4 | 1.5 | Narrowing of colon | 1 | 0.4 |
| Bladder warts | 4 | 1.5 | Bleeding bowel | 1 | 0.4 |
| Bladder gone | 3 | 1.1 | Rest the bowel | 1 | 0.4 |
| Fistula | 3 | 1.1 | Cut away bad waste | 1 | 0.4 |
| Non-malignant growth | 3 | 1.1 | Major operation | 1 | 0.4 |
| Polyposis | 2 | 0.8 | Not told | 33 | 12.5 |
| Bowel lesions | 2 | 0.8 | Can't remember | 3 | 1.1 |
| Move the bowel | 2 | 0.8 | *Total* | 263 | 100.2 |

**Table 4.3**  Cancer patients: recollections of diagnosis

| Recollected diagnosis | n | % |
|---|---|---|
| Cancer | 53 | 31.9 |
| Growth/tumour | 32 | 19.3 |
| Ulcer | 16 | 9.6 |
| Blockage | 12 | 7.2 |
| Remove part of bowel | 7 | 4.2 |
| Polyps | 4 | 2.4 |
| Bladder warts | 4 | 2.4 |
| Abscess | 3 | 1.8 |
| Fistula | 2 | 1.2 |
| Bowel lesions | 2 | 1.2 |
| Move the bowel | 2 | 1.2 |
| Benign cancer | 1 | 0.6 |
| Narrowing of colon | 1 | 0.6 |
| Ulcerative colitis | 1 | 0.6 |
| 2/3 more bowel than most | 1 | 0.6 |
| Sore | 1 | 0.6 |
| Major operation | 1 | 0.6 |
| Bladder infection | 1 | 0.6 |
| Bladder 'gone' | 1 | 0.6 |
| Retention | 1 | 0.6 |
| Not told/can't remember | 20 | 12.0 |
| *Total* | 166 | 99.8 |

that many cancer patients had either not been informed of their actual diagnosis, or did not recall being told about it. However, where these particular patients offered an alternative diagnosis such as 'polyps' or 'ulcer' it seems fairly safe to assume that this was the explanation that was actually given to them. A list of the diagnoses/explanations given to those patients whose actual diagnosis was that of cancer is given in Table 4.3. It is apparent that slightly less than one third of these patients recalled being told their actual diagnosis; approximately one fifth stated that they had a 'growth' or 'tumour' and slightly more than 1 in 10 patients could not remember being told why they had had surgery.

An alternative way of analysing patient responses is related to the degree of specificity about what they recall being told. Accordingly the data were reclassified. Four categories could be clearly distinguished. The first of these includes specific diagnoses, for example cancer, diverticular disease or Crohn's disease. The second includes what might be termed 'lay diagnoses', for example ulcer, perforation or bowel lesions in the absence of any underlying explanation. This category also includes 'growth' or 'tumour' where information relating to malignancy was not given. The third category consists of 'lay explanations' and includes responses such as 'remove part of the bowel', 'need to rest the bowel' and 'bladder gone'. The fourth category includes those patients who did not recall being told about their diagnoses or who stated that they had not been given an explanation. Analysis of patient responses for the whole sample reveals that 38% of patients recalled a specific diagnosis, 39.9% recalled a lay diagnosis, 8.4% a lay explanation and 13.7% could not recall any details.

Why is it that some patients recall more specific details than others? Do surgeons differ in what they tell their patients? Are there patient attributes which have an influence on what they are told? Are there other circumstances which influence the degree to which patients are given a specific diagnosis? Finally, what part do nurses play in giving information to patients?

The literature on this topic would seem to indicate a degree of bias on the part of some authors. For example Elian and Dean (1985) conducted a study of 167 patients who had been suffering from multiple sclerosis for varying lengths of time and report that 83% favoured knowing their diagnosis, 13% were indifferent and fewer than 4% preferred not to know. Yet, 18% of the sample did not know their diagnosis, and it is reported that a large group of the patients had found out this information by accident. Elian and Dean suggest that a policy of non-disclosure is based on a conviction, dogma or emotion and that doctors feel despair and impotence when faced with the incurable patient. On the other hand, Gillon (1985) presents a more balanced viewpoint with arguments both for and against medical paternalism and asks how justifiable it is to add to patients' misery and worry by giving them unpleasant information. Commenting on the study by Elian and Dean, Hopkins (1985) suggests that some patients had been told their diagnosis and had forgotten whereas others may have been consciously, or unconsciously, denying their diagnosis.

In a comprehensive review of the literature McIntosh (1974) raises several important points:

(1) uncertainty of diagnosis or prognosis is one of the main reasons why doctors withold information from patients;

(2) the ideological perspective of doctors who are treating cancer patients may involve judgements about the potential harm in telling or not telling patients about their condition;

(3) the extent of patients' medical knowledge is more important than social class in influencing what doctors tell patients;

(4) 'telling' is not the same as 'communicating' as the latter term implies understanding;

(5) it is not what the patient was told but what he thinks he was told that is important and this may be affected by selective perception and retention of information.

McIntosh also asks how much autonomy a nurse has when it comes to releasing information.

## The surgeon's viewpoint

Interviews with surgeons from the districts taking part in the study support some of the points made by McIntosh. Several surgeons mentioned uncertainty with regard to diagnosis or prognosis. For example:

'I wouldn't be fully frank where I wasn't certain whether I'd cured the condition or not.'

'I don't use the word cancer without a biopsy.'

Sometimes value judgements were also apparent:

'It is unkind to give patients a lot of information that indicates they are going to die rather quickly.'

Patients' medical knowledge also appeared to influence the specificity of what they were told and surgeons often said that the information that they gave was tailored to the individual patient:

'I give as much information as I think they can digest. A lot of patients choose to forget things that they find unpalatable.'

'I use the word 'growth' quite often, expecting the patient to assume that it is malignant and sometimes I'm quite surprised to find that they don't make that assumption.'

This latter example also illustrates the point made by McIntosh, that telling is not the same as communicating which does indeed imply understanding.

## The nursing viewpoint

Many of the ward sisters who were interviewed said that surgeons differed in the extent to which they gave diagnostic details to patients. For example:

'One surgeon is quite candid, he'll say "You've got cancer in your rectum", while others are quite cagey and will say "You've got an ulcer in the back passage", or "You've got a blockage".'

McIntosh raised the question of the autonomy of nurses with regard to giving information to patients. The majority of ward sisters and stoma care nurses who were interviewed in the study had evolved some sort of strategy to deal with this. Whereas giving diagnostic information to patients was the prerogative of the surgeon, sometimes there was an agreement that if patients asked the nurses outright for a diagnosis they had permission to tell them. An alternative strategy would be to bring the patient's request for information to the attention of the surgeon.

Nevertheless, both ward sisters and stoma care nurses often played a major part in clarifying what surgeons had said, explaining the technical details, ensuring that patients understood what they had been told and gauging the extent to which patients were satisfied with the information they had been given. For example:

'I'll say "Are you worried about the ulcer?" or "You think it might be something else?" and quite often patients will say "Well I think I've got cancer." I'll say "Well would you want to know?" and the patient will probably say "No, not as long as they can cure it." Others will say "Yes, I'd like to know and whether I've got rid of it," I then have a word with the surgeon and ask him to have a chat with the patient.'

'The surgeons want me to discuss things with patients. They do the initial telling but sometimes patients ask me and although you don't say exactly the word "cancer" to begin with, you weave a mold around it until they are able to accept the diagnosis.'

'You find that patients reach their own conclusions. They know really inside themselves whether they have got it or they haven't and often nothing is asked and nothing is said but the assumption that we all know what it is just naturally occurs. You find yourself talking about death and about terminal illness without any specific questions having been asked or answered.'

Occasionally, these strategies could break down. One stoma care nurse described how a patient had been told by the surgeon that he had cancer. He then became deeply depressed asking, 'What was all this for?' This particular nurse maintained that a ward sister knows the patients better than the medical staff:

'She can watch his moods and knows what the family have to say. Medical staff should consult the ward sister.'

## The patient's viewpoint

Brewin (1977) describes different types of patients; those who seek reassurance, those who assume an aggressive cheerful optimism and who are upset when given a diagnosis they wish to reject, those who want the full facts, those who don't want to discuss it and live from day to day and those who are tense and suspicious that they are being kept in the dark. Most of these types of reaction were revealed in patient interviews. For example:

'I wanted to know that it was all right but I was frightened to ask if it was.'

'My attitude was—I don't care what you do as long as I know. I've been told everything from the start and that has helped me.'

'I think most people are afraid of the truth, I'd rather carry on from day to day and hope.'

'He didn't say what it was and I didn't ask, the less I know the less I'll have to worry about.'

'He told me that it was a perforated abscess but deep down inside I thought this is just a—I didn't really believe it you know, he was a surgeon.'

There appeared to be several reasons why some patients found it difficult to ask questions. It could be fear of infringing the rules, fear of one's worst suspicions being confirmed, or inability to think of the right questions at the right time. For example:

'You know you can't talk to them when they are busy talking among themselves.'

One patient had not been given the result of a biopsy and was depressed when interviewed:

'I don't know whether I'm allowed to ask what was the result. I thought I would be told whether it was malignant or not but I haven't been told so I'm none the wiser. Whether I am best just keeping quiet I really don't know.'

The comments of another patient illustrate the conflict between wanting to know and being afraid of being told:

'I was terrified inwardly that it was cancer and that I was going to die. I wanted to know that it was all right but I was terrified to ask if it was. You know your mind runs wild. Before I came out of hospital I asked about the results of the tests and all he said was "It was very dangerous but it's OK now". That night I told my husband "I've got cancer and I'm dying"'.

The difficulty of seizing the opportunity of asking questions, particularly in the out-patient department was also amply illustrated:

'You forget when you go and when you get out you think—Oh, I meant to ask. I keep saying I'm going to write a list out next time I go but they haven't time in the out-patients.'

Occasionally patients commented on the way in which surgeons gave them information:

'He told me I'd got a tumour and it would be best to have it done as quickly as possible. I rather got the impression that he thought I knew what was wrong with me, but when I acted in a dismayed manner he sort of back-pedalled.'

'If you asked him a question he somehow managed to politely avoid it. I never got satisfactory answers so I gave up a bit.'

'Everybody begged the question of whether I had a growth there or not, although I knew myself. I suppose I was just trying them out and I was a bit disappointed that nobody thought I would be intelligent enough to be told the truth.'

'This is just what I've picked up you know, listening in and putting two and two together. The doctors use a different language from us don't they?'

## Factors which may influence what patients are told about their diagnosis

### Patient attributes

Further analyses of the data were carried out to see whether the sex or the age of patients might have an influence on what they were told with regard to diagnosis. These analyses showed little difference in specificity between what male and female patients were told. Age differences in the specificity of diagnoses were highly significant for the sample as a whole, but it was thought that this might be due to the effect of including ileostomates who were on average younger and who were more likely to know their diagnosis. Looked at separately, age differences in the specificity of diagnoses were significantly different only for those patients who understood that their stomas were to be temporary, younger patients being more likely to recall a specific diagnosis ($P < 0.05$). A similar trend for those patients with permanent colostomies was not statistically significant.

### Availability of a stoma care nurse and type of admission

The question of whether other circumstances may influence the extent to which patients are given a specific diagnosis was investigated with regard to the type of admission and availability of a stoma care nurse. It would seem possible that patients who are admitted as emergencies may be less likely to be given a specific diagnosis as their preoperative contact is limited. Similarly, as stoma care nurses regard it as part of their role to clarify what surgeons have said, one would expect that patients who had access to a stoma care nurse would be more likely to recall their diagnosis. The percentage of patients who recalled being given a specific diagnosis, a lay diagnosis or a lay explanation or who stated that they were not told or could not remember being told are illustrated for stoma nurse districts and non stoma nurse districts by type of admission in Table 4.4.

The percentages shown in Table 4.4 show that, when all patients in stoma nurse districts are compared to all patients in non stoma nurse districts, there is a trend towards greater specificity in what patients recall being told in non stoma nurse districts. This difference, which is contrary to what might be expected, is not however statistically significant ($\chi^2$ 3 d.f. $= 6.54$).

Table 4.4 also reveals that, if the type of district is ignored and list cases are compared with acute admissions, the difference in what patients recall is statistically significant ($\chi^2$ 2 d.f. $= 6.59$, $P < 0.05$). A greater proportion of patients admitted for elective surgery recall being given a specific diagnosis and a greater proportion of those undergoing emergency surgery either could not recall being told or could not remember what they were told about the

**Table 4.4** Patient recollections: specificity of diagnosis, by type of admission and type of district

| Type of diagnosis | Stoma nurse districts | | | | | | Non stoma nurse districts | | | | | | All districts | | | | | |
|---|---|---|---|---|---|---|---|---|---|---|---|---|---|---|---|---|---|---|
| | Elective | | Acute | | All | | Elective | | Acute | | All | | Elective | | Acute | | All | |
| | n | % | n | % | n | % | n | % | n | % | n | % | n | % | n | % | n | % |
| Specific diagnosis | 55 | 40.7 | 7 | 17.1 | 62 | 35.2 | 29 | 46.0 | 9 | 37.5 | 38 | 43.7 | 84 | 42.4 | 16 | 24.6 | 100 | 38.0 |
| Lay diagnosis | 56 | 41.5 | 22 | 53.7 | 78 | 44.3 | 17 | 27.0 | 10 | 41.7 | 27 | 31.0 | 73 | 36.9 | 32 | 49.2 | 105 | 39.9 |
| Lay explanation | 11 | 8.2 | 0 | 0.0 | 11 | 6.3 | 9 | 14.3 | 2 | 8.3 | 11 | 12.6 | 20 | 10.1 | 2 | 3.1 | 22 | 8.4 |
| Not told/don't know | 13 | 9.6 | 12 | 29.3 | 25 | 14.2 | 8 | 12.7 | 3 | 12.5 | 11 | 12.6 | 21 | 10.6 | 15 | 23.1 | 36 | 13.7 |
| *Total* | 135 | 100.0 | 41 | 100.1 | 176 | 100.0 | 63 | 100.0 | 24 | 100.0 | 87 | 99.9 | 198 | 100.0 | 65 | 100.0 | 263 | 100.0 |

$\chi^2$ 2 d.f. = 8.07, P<0.05 $\qquad$ $\chi^2$ 2 d.f. = 1.83, n.s. $\qquad$ $\chi^2$ 2 d.f. = 6.59, P<0.05

The two smallest categories were combined for analysis

reasons for surgery and what had been done. This difference is in the predicted direction.

However, when list cases are compared with acute admissions separately for stoma nurse districts and non stoma nurse districts, a further surprising finding emerges. It would seem that the difference in specificity of what patients recollect is much greater in stoma nurse districts where, compared with those undergoing elective surgery, far fewer acute admissions recalled specific diagnoses. A majority of patients (53.7%) recalled a lay diagnosis and 29% of patients either could not remember being given a diagnosis or had forgotten what it was ($\chi^2$ 2 d.f. = 8.07, $P < 0.05$). The difference in specificity of what patients were told, according to type of admission was much less in non stoma nurse districts.

## Preoperative preparation

In the course of the interviews, patients were asked whether they had been given any written information during their stay in hospital, who gave them the information and whether they were told what would happen during their stay in hospital.

### Written information

Analysis of responses to the first question revealed very little difference between stoma nurse districts and non stoma nurse districts with regard to the proportion of patients who had been given written information. Approximately three-quarters of the sample had been given a booklet produced by one of the appliance manufacturers or by one of the self-help groups. However, whereas the stoma care nurse was the main provider of written information to those patients who had access to her, patients in the other districts received such information from a variety of sources. Of those patients who did recall being given information one quarter were given booklets by nurses employed by appliance manufacturers, one third received information from nursing staff and one quarter from ward sisters. A few patients were given information by past patients who were themselves ostomates.

Patients were not asked about the quality of the information provided in the booklets, but both favourable and unfavourable comments were sometimes made. Booklets were seen as a valuable source of information but were criticised by a few patients whose experience did not match that described in the text. For example:

'It's roses all the way, isn't it. It gives you a false impression of what is.'

'They say you can eat anything. It's a load of codswallop.'

'In the book it shows a perfectly shaped stoma and it's not like that at all.'

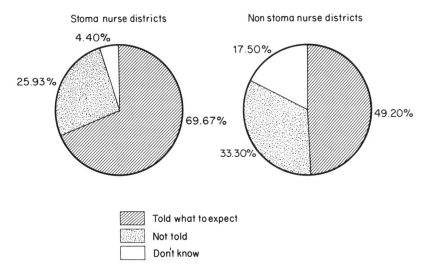

Stoma nurse districts        Non stoma nurse districts

**Figure 4.1**   Percentage of non-acute admissions who recall being told what to expect during their stay in hospital

## Verbal information

The question, 'Were you told what would happen during your stay in hospital?' was confined to those who had undergone elective surgery. Patient responses to this question are given for stoma nurse districts and non stoma nurse districts in Figure 4.1. It can be seen that, whereas more than two-thirds of patients in stoma nurse districts stated that they had been told what to expect, less than one half of the patients in other districts recalled being given this information. This difference is highly significant ($\chi^2$ 2 d.f. = 12.2, $P < 0.01$).

## Postoperative self-care and management of appliances

Another type of information that a patient with a newly-created stoma requires is that which will enable him to cope with his stoma on returning home. For most patients, teaching begins before surgery and continues until discharge. By the time a patient returns home he should know whether he needs to change his diet, how to manage his stoma and that it may change in size or shape. He also needs to know how to obtain and dispose of appliances and what to do if he has any problems or leakage. He should also know of the existence of self-help groups, for example the Colostomy Welfare Association.

The self-care information scale (SCIS), devised to find out whether patients had been given this information and who had given it to them, is described in

**Table 4.5**  Self-care information: means and standard deviations, by type of stoma for stoma nurse and non stoma nurse districts

| Type of stoma | Stoma nurse districts | | | Non stoma nurse districts | | |
|---|---|---|---|---|---|---|
| | n | m | s.d. | n | m | s.d. |
| Permanent colostomy | 69 | 9.6 | 1.66 | 41 | 7.2 | 2.51 |
| Temporary colostomy | 73 | 9.3 | 1.91 | 32 | 6.4 | 3.03 |
| Ileostomy | 17 | 10.3 | 1.6 | 11 | 7.8 | 2.3 |
| Urostomy | 17 | 9.2 | 1.4 | 3 | 8.7 | 2.9 |
| *Total* | 176 | 9.5* | 1.76 | 87 | 7.0* | 2.74 |

* t = 8.82, $P < 0.001$

Chapter 2. It covers items 33–44 in the interview schedule (appendix). The means and standard deviations of scores on this scale are given, separately by type of stoma for each set of districts in Table 4.5. It is immediately apparent that patients from districts where a stoma care nurse was in post had higher scores on this scale. The pattern is consistent for all stoma types but the difference is most marked for those patients who understood that their colostomy might eventually be reversed. The highest SCIS scores were obtained by ileostomates in stoma nurse districts and the lowest scores by temporary colostomates in non stoma nurse districts. The overall difference between SCIS scores for patients, according to whether there was a stoma care nurse available is highly significant (t = 8.86, $P < 0.001$).

In the last chapter we described how almost one half of all temporary colostomates had been admitted for emergency surgery. The means and standard deviations for SCIS scores according to type of district and type of admission are given in Table 4.6. The figures in this table show that, within each set of districts, acute admissions had lower SCIS scores, on average, than those admitted for elective surgery. Over the whole sample, the difference in SCIS scores between those admitted for elective surgery and those admitted for acute surgery is also statistically significant (t = 2.35, $P < 0.05$). However, it can also be seen that acute admissions in stoma nurse districts recalled more

**Table 4.6**  Self-care information scores by type of admission and type of district

| Type of admission | Stoma nurse districts | | | Non stoma nurse districts | | | All districts | | |
|---|---|---|---|---|---|---|---|---|---|
| | n | m | s.d. | n | m | s.d. | n | m | s.d. |
| List | 135 | 9.67 | 1.79 | 63 | 7.17 | 2.73 | 198 | 8.88 | 2.43* |
| Acute | 41 | 8.93 | 1.52 | 24 | 6.63 | 2.76 | 65 | 8.08 | 2.35* |
| *Total* | 176 | 9.50 | 1.76 | 87 | 7.02 | 2.74 | 263 | 8.68 | 2.43 |

* t = 2.35, $P < 0.05$

self-care information than did list cases in districts without stoma nurses and that acute admissions in non stoma nurse districts had the lowest scores. Sex differences in SCIS scores were negligible but SCIS scores were found to be negatively correlated with age; older people tending to recall less information than younger people (r = − 0.26, P < 0.001).

Further differences are apparent when we examine the source of the information given to patients. The percentage of patients who obtained self-care information from different sources in stoma nurse districts is given in Table 4.7. Clearly the stoma care nurse is the main provider of self-care information to patients with other nursing staff involved to a far less extent. There is also evidence of overlap with patients receiving information from more than one source, usually the stoma care nurse and a ward nurse or the ward sister. Ward nurses appear to have been more involved in giving practical advice on stoma care and the changing of appliances than in giving information about other issues, such as the eventual shrinkage of the stoma, obtaining and disposing of used bags and what to do if problems arose after going home.

Considering all sources, it can be seen that the majority of patients recalled being told how to obtain a new supply of appliances, how to dispose of used appliances and what to do if they had problems on returning home. On the other hand, more than a quarter of patients could not recall being told about the different types of appliance that are available and less than half the patients knew about self-help groups. This is somewhat surprising as the addresses of self-help groups are included in the booklets provided.

As a source of information, the booklets do not feature very prominently. However, when the nursing staff had discussed this written material with patients the nurse, and not the booklet, was counted as the source. The figures presented may, therefore, underestimate the importance of this form of information.

The percentage of patients who obtained self-care information from various sources in districts without stoma care nurses is shown in Table 4.8. Clearly, ward nurses are the major source of information for patients in non stoma nurse districts. It is clear that, in these districts also, the nurses concentrate mainly on giving information about the practical aspects of caring for a stoma.

More than one third of patients received a visit from a nurse employed by one or other of the appliance manufacturers. These nurses also provided information to patients, especially about the different types of appliance available, reflecting, possibly, their business interests. Many patients had serious gaps in their knowledge as shown in Table 4.8. For example, 13.8% did not recall being told how to obtain their supply of appliances, 21.8% did not remember being told how to dispose of used bags and 42.5% did not recall being told what to do if they had problems after returning home. Thirty-four per cent did not remember having discussed diet and the same number could

**Table 4.7**  Percentage source of self-care information for patients in stoma nurse districts

| Source of information | How to clean the stoma % | Types of appliance % | How to change the bag % | How often to change the bag % | Disposal % | Supply % | Problems % | Diet % | Remove adhesive % | Shrinkage % | Leakage % | Self-help groups % | All items % |
|---|---|---|---|---|---|---|---|---|---|---|---|---|---|
| Stoma nurse | 76.7 | 66.5 | 76.1 | 71.6 | 79.0 | 89.8 | 88.6 | 67.6 | 74.4 | 62.5 | 44.3 | 26.1 | 68.6 |
| Ward staff | 34.7 | 8.0 | 36.4 | 22.7 | 13.1 | 8.5 | 6.8 | 11.4 | 10.2 | 6.3 | 9.1 | 0.6 | 14.0 |
| Surgeons | – | – | – | – | – | – | 0.6 | 5.7 | – | 3.4 | 0.6 | – | 0.9 |
| Booklet | – | 2.3 | 0.6 | 0.6 | 3.4 | 0.6 | 0.6 | 6.3 | 1.7 | 4.0 | 0.6 | 12.5 | 2.7 |
| Others | 0.6 | 1.1 | 0.6 | 0.6 | – | – | 0.6 | 5.1 | – | – | – | 1.7 | 0.8 |
| Not given | 1.7 | 26.7 | 1.7 | 11.4 | 9.6 | 2.8 | 6.3 | 10.8 | 16.5 | 26.1 | 47.2 | 59.1 | 18.3 |
| *Total* | 113.7* | 104.6 | 114.8 | 106.9 | 105.1 | 101.7 | 103.5 | 106.9 | 1C2.8 | 102.3 | 101.8 | 100.0 | 105.3 |

* Percentages exceed 100 where patients received information from more than one source

**Table 4.8** Percentage source of self-care information for patients in non stoma nurse districts

| Source of information | How to clean the stoma % | Types of appliance % | How to change the bag % | How often to change the bag % | Disposal % | Supply % | Problems % | Diet % | Remove adhesive % | Shrinkage % | Leakage % | Self-help groups % | All items % |
|---|---|---|---|---|---|---|---|---|---|---|---|---|---|
| Stoma nurse from elsewhere | 1.1 | 1.1 | 2.3 | 2.3 | 2.3 | 1.1 | 1.1 | 1.1 | – | 3.4 | – | – | 1.2 |
| Ward staff | 79.3 | 27.6 | 80.5 | 47.1 | 55.2 | 64.4 | 35.6 | 36.8 | 31.0 | 43.7 | 14.9 | 13.8 | 43.9 |
| Surgeons | – | – | – | – | – | – | 1.1 | 6.9 | – | 1.1 | – | 1.1 | 0.9 |
| Booklet | 2.3 | 2.3 | – | – | 8.0 | 3.4 | 2.3 | 6.9 | 1.1 | 5.7 | – | 8.0 | 3.4 |
| Company nurse | 10.3 | 19.5 | 9.2 | 10.3 | 10.3 | 13.8 | 14.9 | 10.3 | 8.0 | 10.3 | 4.6 | 9.2 | 11.1 |
| Others | 1.1 | 5.7 | 1.1 | 1.1 | 3.4 | 3.4 | 2.3 | 4.6 | 3.4 | 2.3 | 1.1 | 11.5 | 3.8 |
| Not given | 9.2 | 44.8 | 10.3 | 41.4 | 21.8 | 13.8 | 42.5 | 34.5 | 57.5 | 34.5 | 80.5 | 59.8 | 37.4 |
| *Total* | 103.3 | 101.0 | 103.4 | 102.2 | 101.0 | 99.9 | 99.8 | 101.0 | 101.0 | 101.0 | 101.1 | 103.4 | 101.7 |

not recall being told that their stoma would probably become smaller and that they might then need a different size of appliance.

As in stoma nurse districts, less than one half of these patients remembered being told about self-help groups. Similarly, the booklets do not appear to have been a major source of information.

### Patient satisfaction with information

The findings with regard to three types of information have been presented; those relating to diagnosis, preoperative preparation and postoperative self care/management of appliances. In the framework for evaluation (Chapter 1), we concluded that the kind of information given was perhaps less important than patient satisfaction with the information given. Certainly, the findings relating to diagnosis suggest that not all patients wish to know the full details of their illness. In order to gauge the extent of satisfaction, patients were asked if, on looking back, there was anything else that they would have liked to have been told. The responses to this question are shown, separately, for the two sets of districts in Figure 4.2.

Three-quarters of the total sample said that there was nothing more that they would have liked to have been told and one fifth of all the patients interviewed would have liked more information. The percentage of patients who were dissatisfied with the information given is larger in non stoma nurse districts; more than one quarter of these patients would have liked more

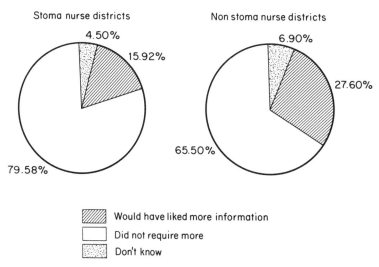

**Figure 4.2**   Percentage of patients who would have liked more information

**Table 4.9**  Specificity of diagnosis (and number of patients), by desire for more information

|  | Specific diagnosis (n = 100) % | Lay diagnosis (n = 105) % | Lay explanation (n = 22) % | Not told/ can't remember (n = 36) % |
|---|---|---|---|---|
| Would have liked more information | 31.0 | 14.3 | 13.6 (3) | 8.3 (3) |
| Did not require more information | 64.0 | 82.9 | 86.4 (19) | 75.0 (27) |
| Don't know | 5.0 | 2.9 | 0.0 | 16.7 (6) |
| *Total* | 100.0 | 100.1 | 100.0 | 100.0 |

information. The difference between the two sets of districts is statistically significant ($\chi^2$ 2 df. = 6.12, $P < 0.05$).

While there was little difference between the sexes with regard to the desire for more information, there was a tendency for those who would have liked more information to be younger and for those who said that they 'didn't know' to be older. These differences are not statistically significant.

Somewhat surprisingly, it would seem that the proportion of patients who would have liked more information is greater for those who recalled a specific diagnosis and declines progressively according to the level of specificity of diagnostic details recalled (Table 4.9). So what was it that patients would have liked to have been told? The interview transcripts revealed a variety of responses. These have been classified according to content under six headings and are shown, separately for the two sets of districts, in Table 4.10.

Evidently there was no single source of dissatisfaction. As a percentage of the whole sample of patients, only 6.8% stated that they would have liked more information relating to diagnosis or explanation of the surgical procedure. Some of these are worthy of note. For example, two patients did

**Table 4.10**  Information patients would have liked to have been given, by type of district

|  | Stoma nurse districts (n = 176) % | Non stoma nurse districts (n = 87) % | All (n = 263) % |
|---|---|---|---|
| Surgical/diagnostic details | 6.8 | 6.9 | 6.8 |
| Appliances/care of stoma | 1.7 | 8.0 | 3.8 |
| Physical after-effects | 2.3 | 3.4 | 2.7 |
| Practical advice/sources of advice | 1.1 | 4.6 | 2.3 |
| Emotional after-effects | 0.6 | 2.3 | 1.1 |
| Tests/examinations/tubes/drains | 1.1 | 1.1 | 1.1 |
| Everything/general explanation | 2.3 | 1.1 | 1.9 |
| *Total* | 15.9 | 27.4 | 19.8 |

not know that they had had excision of rectum. The wife of one of these patients thought that the wound was a bedsore. Two other patients did not know whether their bladder had been removed. Other patients would have liked to have been told whether their tumour was malignant, how deep it was or whether there was a recurrence. Others would have liked to have been told what the operation entailed. (It is also worth noting here that, when asked earlier in the interview if their stoma was permanent or temporary, 14% of colostomates who had not had excision of the rectum said that they didn't know.)

Some patients would have liked to have had more information about stoma care appliances, what was available, how to obtain equipment, how often to change their bag or how to reduce odour problems. The percentage of patients requiring this knowledge was higher in non stoma nurse districts (8%), than in stoma nurse districts (1.7%).

Physical after-effects, such as having a bowel action (temporary ostomates), pain, healing time and weight were mentioned by a minority of patients. Emotional after-effects, or how to come to terms with life with a stoma were also mentioned by a minority of patients.

Although only three patients stated that they would have liked to have been told beforehand about tests, examinations or drips and drains, approximately 1 in 10 patients, some of whom had been prepared to expect this, mentioned the proliferation of tubing and/or discomfort from drips or drains after surgery. For example:

'I felt grotesque: like a monster.'

'Tubes everywhere, I felt like an old man.'

A few patients (2.3%) stated that they would have liked to have been given more practical advice, for example, what to eat or what not to eat, how much exercise they could take or whom to approach for practical advice on returning home.

Five patients could not specify what it was that they would have liked to have been told:

'Everything. I didn't grasp it.'

## Discussion

Taken at face value, it would seem that, whereas a minority of patients (38%) recalled being given a specific diagnosis, the majority of patients were satisfied with the information received. However, there are several anomalies in the data which remain unexplained. For example, proportionately fewer patients in stoma nurse districts recalled a specific diagnosis but proportionately more patients appeared to be satisfied when compared to patients in other districts.

One possible explanation for this is that the efforts made by stoma care nurses to clarify what surgeons had said led to greater recall of lay diagnoses and/or greater satisfaction.

There is a further anomaly in that, compared with patients in other districts, patients in stoma nurse districts who were admitted for emergency surgery were less likely to recall a specific diagnosis. Indeed a greater proportion of these patients were unable to remember what, if anything, they had been told about their illness. The reasons for this are open to conjecture. One possible, but not entirely convincing, explanation is that surgeons who are on call are more inclined to leave explanations, including diagnosis, to the stoma care nurse when one is available. Whatever the explanation, it would appear that these patients are less well informed and that the strategy described by nurses to ensure that patients are given the information they need, may not always work.

Interpretation of the finding that a greater proportion of patients who recalled their diagnosis would have liked additional information is also somewhat difficult. It would appear that those who are keen to be informed are being given more specific information; their needs are being recognised. It may simply be, as Cohen and Lazarus (1982) suggest, that some patients are insatiable in their search for information. Cohen and Lazarus refer to two studies which investigated the relationship between recovery from surgery and avoidance or vigilance toward seeking information about the medical condition and surgery. Both studies showed that those who knew the most about their operations had the slowest and most complicated recovery (Cohen and Lazarus, 1973; Cohen, 1975). The authors suggest that 'vigilant copers' seek to master the world by seeking information but that this style is maladaptive in the postoperative period when people are relatively powerless. If they are correct in their hypothesis then it may be that questions relating to satisfaction with information may be tapping a dimension of personality. An alternative hypothesis is that patients who experience greater suffering tend to seek more information about their condition and do less well postoperatively because they were more ill to begin with. Whatever the explanation, patient satisfaction would appear to be an important variable which will be further explored in later analyses.

A further complication arises from the fact that the findings presented in this study are based on patient recall. Undoubtedly, with a sample of mainly elderly patients, some will forget what they have been told. It may be that they tend to forget the label rather than the explanations that they were given so that fewer patients recall specific diagnoses. Unfortunately, it is not easy to distinguish between lapses of memory and conscious or unconscious denial. The finding that 38% of patients recalled a specific diagnosis is almost certainly an underestimate of the proportion of patients who were given their actual diagnosis. For example, Bond (1983) was a participant observer over a 12-month period on two wards. She describes the different coping strategies employed by cancer patients, some of whom sought diagnostic and prognostic information while others engaged in selective information seeking and avoidance and rationalisation as methods of coping. Bond suggests that staff did not take account of these different strategies but sought to avoid reference to cancer or its implications. The finding in this study, that fewer cancer patients recalled a specific diagnosis, probably reflects both greater use of euphemisms by surgeons and selective retention and denial by patients.

A more detailed study of patient satisfaction with information reported by Engstrom (1984) yielded much higher levels of dissatisfaction than those found in this study. Engstrom reports that, out of a sample of 95 patients, 31 said that they had received no information relating to diagnosis (32.6%). This figure is much higher than the 13.3% of patients in this study who could not recall being told anything about their need for surgery. However, it seems probable that the difference in findings is compounded by differences in the methods used. In this study patients were asked, in face-to-face interview, why they had the operation and what they were told. They were also asked whether there was anything else that they would have liked to have been told and, if so, what this was. The patients interviewed by Engstrom were not all surgical patients, they had been sent the information scales beforehand and had time to ponder their answers before being interviewed by telephone. Locker and Dunt (1978) suggest that individuals may report satisfaction or dissatisfaction with particular aspects of care when asked directly, but may not give sufficient priority to these aspects to mention them spontaneously in response to an open-ended question. Clearly, there is a need for exploration of differences related to the methods used if we wish to be more sure of the validity of our findings.

The results relating to preoperative preparation and self-care information before discharge are much easier to interpret. It is quite clear that patients who are admitted for elective surgery are not only better informed about their diagnosis but that they also have greater knowledge of self-care before being discharged from hospital. It is also quite clear that patients in stoma nurse districts were much better informed than patients in other districts who received information from a variety of sources including, in some cases, nurses employed by appliance manufacturers. Indeed, by the time patients were interviewed, at approximately 10 weeks following surgery, 60% of patients in non stoma nurse districts had seen a company nurse at some time or other. This contact will be explored more fully in the next chapter which looks at patients' experience in hospital.

## Summary

(1) Less than one third of cancer patients recalled being told that they had cancer.

(2) Over the whole sample, 38% of patients recalled a specific diagnosis, 40% recalled a lay diagnosis, 8% a lay explanation of the reason for surgery and 14% could not recall any details.

(3) Compared with patients in stoma nurse districts, a higher percentage of patients who did not have access to a stoma care nurse recalled being given a specific diagnosis.

(4) A greater proportion of patients admitted for elective surgery recalled a specific diagnosis compared with acute admissions of whom almost one quarter could not recall being told their diagnosis. This difference was most marked in the districts that employed stoma care nurses.

(5) Approximately three-quarters of the sample had been given written information relating to stoma care.

(6) More than two-thirds of patients in stoma nurse districts, but less than half of patients in non stoma nurse districts, said that they had been told what to expect during their stay in hospital.

(7) Scores on the self-care information scale (SCIS) were significantly higher for patients in stoma nurse districts than for patients in other districts where temporary ostomates or acute admissions had the lowest scores.

(8) In non stoma nurse districts 14% of patients did not recall being told how to obtain their supply of appliances before being discharged. Twenty-two per cent of patients did not recall being told how to dispose of used appliances and 43% did not recall being told what to do if they had problems after returning home.

(9) One fifth of the sample stated that they would have liked more information, the proportion being significantly greater for patients in non stoma nurse districts.

# 5

# Patients' Hospital Experience

'I'm no longer the woman I used to be,
They've put me together quite differently.'

### Siting of the stoma

Many stoma care nurses consider the careful siting of a stoma to be an essential part of their role. Accordingly, patients were asked whether anyone had marked their abdomen or placed a bag in position before surgery and, if so, who did this. Their responses are summarised, by type of admission, for the two sets of districts in Table 5.1. In compiling this table it was assumed that, when no-one had marked the site of the stoma beforehand, the site was determined later by the surgeon.

It can be seen that in stoma nurse districts one third of the patients had their stomas sited by stoma care nurses alone. A minority of stomas were sited by the stoma care nurse and surgeon together but surgeons were assumed to be responsible in 60.7% of cases. Involvement of stoma care nurses in this aspect of care was minimal when patients were admitted for emergency surgery.

In non stoma nurse districts, company nurses or ward sisters sited a few stomas, but the majority were positioned by the surgeon.

In the interviews that were held later, surgeons and nursing staff were asked who sited stomas. In non stoma nurse districts there was evidence of the increasing involvement of ward sisters. In two districts, the ward sisters who were interviewed had recently completed stoma care courses and were now siting stomas. A company nurse was involved in one district only and in a further two districts the positioning of stomas was said to be a team decision. It was also considered to be a team decision in three of the stoma nurse districts. Stoma care nurses were said to be responsible for siting stomas on behalf of the majority of surgeons in seven districts. Staff, in one district only, said that the surgeon made the decision. This particular question gave rise to several comments especially from ward sisters. For example:

**Table 5.1** Who determined the site of the stoma, by type of district and type of admission

| | Stoma nurse districts | | | Non stoma nurse districts | | | All | | |
| | List (n=135) % | Acute (n=41) % | All (n=176) % | List (n=63) % | Acute (n=24) % | All (n=87) % | List (n=198) % | Acute (n=65) % | All (n=263) % |
|---|---|---|---|---|---|---|---|---|---|
| Surgeon | 60.7 | 97.6 | 69.3 | 93.6 | 91.7 | 93.1 | 71.2 | 95.4 | 77.2 |
| Stoma care nurse | 33.3 | 0.0 | 25.6 | 0.0 | 0.0 | 0.0 | 22.7 | 0.0 | 17.1 |
| Surgeon and stoma care nurse | 5.2 | 2.4 | 4.5 | 0.0 | 0.0 | 0.0 | 3.5 | 1.5 | 3.0 |
| Company nurse | 0.0 | 0.0 | 0.0 | 3.2 | 4.2 | 3.4 | 1.0 | 1.5 | 1.1 |
| Ward sister | 0.7 | 0.0 | 0.6 | 3.2 | 4.2 | 3.4 | 1.5 | 1.5 | 1.5 |
| Total | 99.9 | 100.0 | 100.0 | 100.0 | 100.1 | 99.9 | 99.9 | 99.9 | 99.9 |

'It is usually done by the surgeon with the patient on the operating table so you can imagine the problems that that entails.'

'The stoma organised by the stoma nurse is far superior. The stomas created in emergency surgery are often more difficult. They are always far too near the wounds or far too near the rib cage when the patient is sitting up.'

However, one of the surgeons interviewed also had a comment to make:

'The stoma nurse [marks the site] and then we always move it by a centimetre just to make sure that we are independent!'

Of course, for various reasons, there is no guarantee that a stoma will actually be placed where the site has been marked but is there any evidence to suggest that stomas which have been sited by nursing staff are easier to manage? One criterion is that patients should be able to see their stomas easily and this question was put to them in interview. Their responses are given, according to who sited the stoma by type of admission in Table 5.2.

It might be expected that the stomas of patients undergoing elective surgery would be superior in terms of ease of visibility compared to those stomas created in acute surgery. Taking the sample as a whole, this was found to be the case, but the difference is marginal; 86.9% of list cases and 81.5% of acute admissions said that they could see their stomas easily. In order to compare stomas sited by surgeons with those sited by stoma care nurses it is necessary to look at list cases only. It was found that of those sited by surgeons 84.4% were easily visible to the patient compared with 92% of those sited by nurses. This difference is not statistically significant ($\chi^2$ 2 d.f. = 2.64) but might be considered highly significant from the patients' point of view. The figures just quoted sound quite high but they also imply that, over the whole sample approximately 1 in 7 patients had difficulty in seeing their stomas. Many of these patients said that they used a mirror when changing their appliance but in the worst cases even this did not help. Comments from patients illustrated the problems caused by badly sited stomas which made bending difficult, were too near the navel causing leakage, too close to the hip bone or were no longer visible now that they had regained weight.

### Reaction to the stoma

The profusion of papers written about the implications of a change in body image would lead us to suspect that, for the majority of patients, stoma surgery is devastating and that the first sight of a new stoma is a traumatic experience for most patients. Indeed, Morrow (1976) suggests that patients are almost universally shocked to see the stoma postoperatively and Druss et al (1969) report that two-thirds of a sample of 36 colostomates described an unpleasant initial reaction.

The implications of this for nursing appear to be threefold. First, it would

**Table 5.2** Patient ability to see the stoma, by who determined the site and type of admission

| | Sited by surgeon only | | | Sited by nurses only | | | All[1] | | |
|---|---|---|---|---|---|---|---|---|---|
| | List (n=141) % | Acute (n=62) % | All (n=203) % | List (n=50) % | Acute (n=2) % | All (n=52) % | List (n=198) % | Acute (n=65) % | All (n=263) % |
| Able to see stoma easily | 84.4 | 80.6 | 83.3 | 92.0 | (2) | 92.3 | 86.9 | 81.5 | 85.6 |
| Unable to see stoma easily | 15.6 | 19.4 | 16.7 | 6.0 | (0) | 5.8 | 12.6 | 18.5 | 14.1 |
| Don't know | 0.0 | 0.0 | 0.0 | 2.0 | (0) | 1.9 | 0.5 | 0.0 | 0.4 |
| *Total* | 100.0 | 100.0 | 100.0 | 100.0 | (2) | 100.0 | 100.0 | 100.0 | 100.1 |

[1] Eight patients, whose stomas were sited by surgeons and nurses together, are included here. Approximately half of those who could not see the stoma easily used a mirror

seem important that the patient is thoroughly prepared so that the initial shock is reduced. This preparation includes teaching the patient about the construction of a stoma, how it will function and what it will look like both postoperatively and at a later stage when it has settled down. Second, it is important that the patient is psychologically prepared before seeing the stoma. This entails giving reassurance and choosing an appropriate time. Third, when the bag is being changed by the nurse postoperatively, she must not give any indication of feelings of revulsion because the patient will be watching her face carefully (Black, 1985). Indeed, Abrams (1984) maintains that nurses need to evaluate their own feelings towards abdominal stomas if they are to give the best possible care.

Accordingly, in the later interviews with nursing staff, we asked who was usually present when a patient saw his stoma for the first time. The most common reply received from ward sisters in non stoma nurse districts was that it could be any of the nursing staff. Two ward sisters elaborated on this theme. The first said that patients were never made to look at their stomas or change their bags until they decided that they were ready to do so, and the second described how staff gradually introduced the patient to the new stoma:

'We get patients used to looking at it while watching what we are doing. I don't like nurses wearing gloves for this kind of thing because it puts a barrier there in the patient's mind. If they see that we treat it as perfectly normal they will.'

When this question was asked in stoma nurse districts, the most common response was that the stoma care nurse was usually present when a patient looked at the stoma for the first time. When this was not possible the ward sister or trained staff were more likely to be there. Several stoma care nurses elaborated on the importance of adequate preparation beforehand. With regard to acute admissions one stoma care nurse said:

'You have to spend a lot longer with a patient like that because you have to calm him down. If patients are not prepared it is more difficult for them.'

Another stoma care nurse described how, once patients knew exactly what the stoma would look like and how it would function, she would show the stoma to patients through the bag. Another of these nurses also commented on the importance of the nurse's attitude:

'I believe that most patients do not look at the stoma when an appliance is changed, they look at whoever is removing the appliance to see how the nurse reacts and if the nurse reacts OK they will look then.'

Patients were asked three questions relating to seeing the stoma for the first time:

(1) When did you first look at your stoma?

(2) How did you feel when you first saw your stoma?

(3) Were you reluctant to look at it at first?

Only 3% of patients had not looked at their stoma before discharge and a further 2% first saw the stoma after transferring to another hospital for convalescence. One patient emphasised that, although he had seen his stoma he had not actually 'looked' at it. When asked how they felt, patients responded in many different ways:

'I thought "My God! I would rather have had my legs taken".'

'I was shocked to the marrow, said I'd never forgive the doctor for that.'

'It is unnatural to wake up in hospital and find that your body's been altered. It's something that I've had done to me which I had no control over.'

'I had no idea what to expect.'

'It wasn't as bad as I expected, it looked just as it should be, a natural part of the body in fact.'

'Fascinating really, I was just glad because of all the pain I'd been having.'

The responses of patients were subsequently grouped by two researchers into five categories ranging from very positive affect to very negative affect:

(1) amused/glad/marvellous;

(2) not bothered/not worried, accepted it;

(3) apathetic, didn't care/forgotten, mixed feelings/indifferent;

(4) afraid, difficult to accept, worried, a bit upset;

(5) terrified/sick/shocked/ashamed/disgust/mutilated/hated it/cried.

The distribution of responses between these five categories is given, by type of stoma, in Figure 5.1. Just over a half of the total sample of patients expressed positive affect and one third of the patients reported extremely negative reactions. These figures compare favourably with those reported by Druss et al (1969). In accordance with the notion of 'trade off' (Chapter 1), it can also be seen that a greater proportion of ileostomates reported a positive reaction. Compared with other ostomates those with a urinary stoma expressed more negative affect and a greater proportion of temporary colostomates reported negative affect when compared with permanent colostomates. Although these differences were to be expected, they are not statistically significant. There was very little difference in reported affect for patients in the two sets of districts but a greater proportion of women expressed negative affect than the men. Whereas more than one half of the male sample reported positive affect (58%), more than one half of all females reported a negative reaction when looking at the stoma for the first time (52.5%). This difference is statistically significant ($\chi^2$ 4 d.f. = 13.3, $P < 0.01$)

A further difference was found when acute admissions were compared with those undergoing elective surgery. This difference is also in the expected

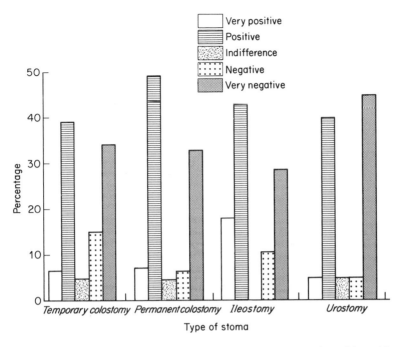

**Figure 5.1**    Reactions to the stoma. Percentage of patients responding with positive or negative affect, by type of stoma

direction; a greater proportion of acute admissions reporting negative affect ($\chi^2$ 4 d.f. $= 10.58$, $P < 0.05$).

Analysis of these data by age revealed a slight trend for older patients to report positive initial reactions to the stoma more frequently than younger patients. This trend was not statistically significant.

### Involvement of family/spouse

The importance of family involvement in the rehabilitation of the ostomate has also been discussed in Chapter 1. Accordingly, patients were asked whether anyone in their family had been given information about the care of their stoma. If patients said 'No' they were then asked whether they would have liked this. Responses to these questions are given in Figure 5.2 for the two sets of districts.

We can see that family involvement was very much greater for patients in stoma nurse districts where almost one half of patients said that a family member had been given information relating to stoma care. In contrast, a greater proportion of patients from non stoma nurse districts said that they

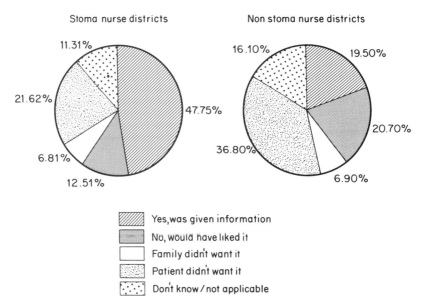

**Figure 5.2** Percentage of patients whose family was given information about caring for the stoma

would have liked information to be given to a member of their family and a greater proportion of patients said that they had not wanted this. These differences are in the predicted direction and are highly significant ($\chi^2$ 4 d.f. $= 20.65$, $P < 0.001$). There was little difference between the sexes on this question.

Several patients mentioned being apprehensive about the reaction of their spouse to the stoma. For example:

> 'I thought it might put . . . off but anyway sister talked to him and showed him and explained it all and he took it very well really. Oh, it worried me I'll tell you. I could have wept buckets.'

> 'At one time I thought my husband would be appalled by it but I think it's me that was appalled by it more.'

## Management of appliances

Patients were also asked whether they had had any practice in changing their appliance before being discharged and, if so, whether they felt that this was sufficient. Responses to these questions are illustrated in Figure 5.3 for the two sets of districts. Taking the sample as a whole, 1 in 10 patients said that they had had no practice in changing their appliance before going home, and approximately 1 in 10 patients felt that they had not had enough practice.

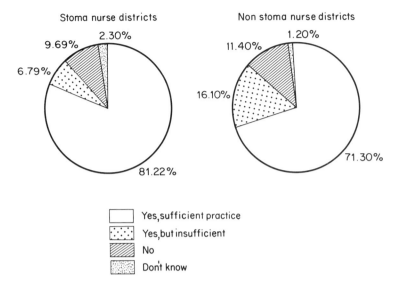

Figure 5.3 cont.

**Figure 5.3**  Percentage of patients who had practice in changing their appliance before discharge

Although there is little difference in the overall proportion of patients who had practice in changing their appliance before discharge, the proportion of patients who felt that this was insufficient was greater in non stoma nurse districts. This difference is in the predicted direction and is statistically significant ($\chi^2$ 2 d.f. = 5.83, $P < 0.05$).

## Visitors in hospital

Details were taken of the visitors received by the patients.

### Stoma care nurses

In stoma nurse districts, only one patient reported that he had not seen a stoma care nurse. The great majority of patients said that they found these visits helpful. In the other districts no-one saw a stoma care nurse during their stay in hospital.

### Company nurses

In contrast, none of the patients in stoma nurse districts said that they had been visited by a company nurse during their hospital stay but 41% of patients in other districts said that they had been seen by a company nurse and most of them said that they had found this helpful.


## Social workers

Almost 1 in 5 patients had been visited by a social worker and there was little difference between the two sets of districts with regard to these visits. Although they were largely seen as helpful there were exceptions. For example, one patient was asked by a social worker if she felt degraded after having stoma surgery. The patient reported that following this she began to wonder if she did.


## General practitioners

Over the whole sample less than 1 in 10 patients received a visit from their GP. These visits were generally appreciated and 15% of patients said that they would have liked a visit. The remainder didn't feel that it was necessary.


## Established ostomates

Ward sisters and stoma care nurses were asked whether they invited established ostomates to visit stoma patients. With the exception of two districts there appeared to be a common policy of asking patients if they would like to talk to someone with an established stoma and, if the patient wished to do so, attempts would be made to match the patient for age, sex and lifestyle. In the two districts that did not follow this policy, one had a stoma care nurse who was herself an ostomate. The ward sister in the other district that did not have a stoma care nurse said that she had never had anyone who was willing to do these visits. One ward sister said that patients whose stomas were deemed to be temporary were not asked if they would like a visit.

Only one ward sister said that she used a self-help group to supply visitors. Two of the stoma care nurses stipulated that they did not use official visitors following very unfortunate experiences by their patients.

Most staff also said that patients often did not wish to see anyone in the postoperative period but that they might change their minds later and a visit could then be arranged. One stoma care nurse said that, whereas ileostomates almost always wished to speak to someone else with an established stoma, colostomates almost always did not wish to do so.

Patients were asked if anyone who had had stoma surgery in the past, had come to see them. Fewer than 1 in 5 patients said that they had seen such a person, but most of those who had said that they had found the visit helpful.

There was little difference between the two sets of districts with regard to the frequency of these visits but proportionately more ileostomates had received visits than patients with other types of stoma and 'temporary' ostomates had been visited least.

More than one third of those who had not seen an established ostomate said that they would have liked to have been able to talk to someone with an established stoma. These findings are in agreement with those of Mitchell (1980) who, reporting a survey of stoma care in Scotland, said that the majority of colostomates visited in hospital felt better as a result of a visit from a patient who had recovered from stoma surgery. Trainor (1982) suggests that serving in the visitor role contributes to predicting a higher level of acceptance of ostomy. If this is so, then these visits could be mutually beneficial.

## Overview of hospital experience

Towards the end of the interview, patients were asked whether any one person had been particularly helpful while they were in hospital. The percentage responses to this question are given separately for the two sets of districts in Table 5.3.

It can be seen that, in non stoma nurse districts, ward nursing staff were more frequently seen as having been particularly helpful than any other person or group. Of those who said that no one person had been particularly helpful many said that everyone had been helpful.

**Table 5.3** The percentage of people said to be particularly helpful to patients during their stay in hospital, by type of district

|  | Stoma nurse districts (n = 176) % | Non stoma nurse districts (n = 87) % |
| --- | --- | --- |
| Ward nursing staff | 26.7 | 40.9 |
| Stoma care nurse | 18.8 | 0.0 |
| Relatives/friends | 10.8 | 13.8 |
| Surgeon | 10.2 | 2.3 |
| Other hospital staff | 1.1 | 3.4 |
| Company nurse | 0.0 | 1.1 |
| Established ostomate | 0.6 | 0.0 |
| Another patient | 0.0 | 1.1 |
| Patient himself | 0.0 | 1.1 |
| No one person particularly helpful | 35.3 | 36.3 |
| *Total* | 103.5* | 100.0 |

* Some patients cited more than one person

Although ward nursing staff were cited less frequently by patients in stoma nurse districts, they still feature more prominently than the stoma care nurse. This may be taken to indicate that having access to a stoma care nurse does not entirely detract from the role of ward staff in caring for the patient with a new stoma.

Interestingly, relatives and friends were mentioned by more than 1 in 10 patients overall, thus emphasising the value of family involvement in patient care.

### Hospital memories

Finally, we asked the question:

> 'Apart from the actual operation is there anything about your stay in hospital that particularly stands out in your memory?'

Responses to this question were grouped under several headings. A very similar pattern emerged for the two sets of districts and the percentages for the whole sample are given in Table 5.4.

Approximately twice as many patients said that their most outstanding memory was of good care or good ward conditions than of poor care or poor ward conditions. Praise was given to the devotion, kindness, humour or tenacity of staff and some praised the food and comfort of the ward. Indeed, one patient likened the ward to a 'seven-star hotel' and another said that 'he'd had a damn good holiday'! However, there were also criticisms, such as delay in answering calls, inexperience of staff, unhygienic practices and lack of

**Table 5.4**   Memories of hospital stay: percentage responses

|  | Whole sample (n = 263) % |
| --- | --- |
| Good care | 27.8 |
| Good ward conditions | 4.9 |
| Poor care | 9.1 |
| Poor ward conditions | 8.0 |
| Treatment related | 9.1 |
| Physical problems | 7.6 |
| Interpersonal events | 5.3 |
| Stoma related events | 3.0 |
| Loneliness/depression | 2.3 |
| Extraordinary events | 1.9 |
| Nothing particularly | 20.9 |
| *Total* | 99.9 |

information. Hard beds or pillows, lack of privacy, noise and poor food were also criticised.

The physical problems which patients remembered included postoperative confusion and hallucinations, pain, retention of urine and discomfort on sitting (sometimes for long periods).

A small percentage of patients had, as their most outstanding memory, the help they had received from other patients or the suffering of others.

Almost 1 in 10 patients recalled discomfort caused by tests, drips, drains or injections. For a minority of patients, their most outstanding memory was of feeling depressed or lonely.

Although the stoma was mentioned by only a few, the experience of one patient is worth recounting in the hope that such an occurrence may be prevented in the future:

'One night I started to move around the ward and go to the day room and suddenly I felt something run into the bag rather freely. I covered it with my hand and I could feel it warm and swelling rather rapidly. I retreated to the ward and the night staff hadn't long come on and I said to the staff nurse, "Staff, I'm filling up rapidly here, I wonder if you could help me" because I wasn't at the stage of changing my bag or emptying my bag. She said "OK . . . I'll be back in a moment". She had a gentleman who was dying a few rooms down and there was a lady on the other side of the ward experiencing something of a crisis. So she dashed off and came back 20 minutes later and I said "Staff, it's critical now". "Right", she said, "I'm coming". But with that there was a terrific bursting, the whole thing burst off and this horrible, foul smelling, I don't know it couldn't just be body, stomach muck, it must have been chemicals that had been pumped into me for weeks and just fell all over the place and she said "Don't panic". And it spouted like a water spout, all over the floor and she said, "Ah well, you missed the bed, that's the important thing". I was frightened, I was scared and I could see she was too but she wasn't supposed to show she was. So she said "Hold on" and while she turned her back it started again. And that is when I saw her being very, very concerned. There seemed to be no stopping to it so she grabbed hold of, I don't know, an old pair of pyjamas or something and just sort of covered the thing. I stood there and all I wanted to do was to cry. I'd never felt such utter despair in all my life. That was a real low point for me, that is one experience I shall never forget.'

At 10 weeks after surgery, this patient had no confidence in his appliance and was acutely anxious about returning to hospital for a reversal of his stoma. Unfortunately, this was not the only incidence of bags bursting or blowing off while patients were still in hospital although it is certainly the most horrific.

## Postoperative length of stay

Clearly, some patients take longer than others to recover from surgery. Patients also vary in the length of time required to learn how to cope with a stoma. Given that we might expect these variations, is it possible that having access to a stoma care nurse affects the postoperative length of stay in hospital and do districts differ in their policy with regard to the discharge of patients following stoma surgery?

In seeking answers to these questions, we need to take account of the availability of convalescent beds as this might contribute to earlier discharge. Accordingly, postoperative days spent in hospital were combined with days spent in a convalescent home/hospital for the purpose of analysis.

Over the whole sample of 263 patients the average postoperative length of stay in hospital/convalescent home was 22.8 days. As expected there was a large variation ranging from 7 to 88 days. For those who had abdomino-perineal excision of the rectum the average postoperative length of stay was 23.3 days, for those whose colostomy was deemed temporary it was 26 days, for ileostomates it was 26 days and for urostomates it was 19.7 days.

Eighteen per cent of patients spent an average of 13.3 days in either a convalescent home or outlying hospital. These patients were distributed over 10 districts, but extensive use of convalescent beds was evident in only two districts (one of which had a stoma care nurse in post). Thus, there was little difference in the use of convalescent beds between the two sets of districts.

The average length of time spent in hospital/convalescent home by patients in stoma nurse districts was 22.1 days and ranged from 7 to 80 days. The average for patients in non stoma nurse districts was 24.1 days and ranged from 7 to 88 days. The discharge pattern, over time, for the two sets of districts is shown in Table 5.5.

It can be seen that 60.3% of patients in stoma nurse districts were discharged in less than 3 weeks compared with 45.9% of patients in non stoma nurse districts. Thereafter, the discrepancy becomes smaller. When the figures for each district are compared, there appears to be a distinct trend for patients

**Table 5.5** Discharge patterns for patients in districts with and districts without stoma care nurses

| Days postoperative | Districts with stoma care nurse (n = 176) | | Districts without stoma care nurse (n = 87) | | All | |
|---|---|---|---|---|---|---|
| | % | Cumulative % | % | Cumulative % | % | Cumulative % |
| 7–10 | 6.3 | 6.3 | 8.0 | 8.0 | 6.8 | 6.8 |
| 11–15 | 33.0 | 39.3 | 24.1 | 32.1 | 30.0 | 36.8 |
| 16–20 | 21.0 | 60.3 | 13.8 | 45.9 | 18.6 | 55.4 |
| 21–25 | 9.7 | 70.0 | 17.2 | 63.1 | 12.2 | 67.6 |
| 26–30 | 13.1 | 83.1 | 17.2 | 80.3 | 14.5 | 82.1 |
| 31–35 | 6.8 | 89.9 | 5.8 | 86.1 | 6.5 | 88.6 |
| 36–40 | 2.8 | 92.7 | 3.4 | 89.5 | 3.0 | 91.6 |
| 41–45 | 1.1 | 93.8 | 1.2 | 90.7 | 1.1 | 92.7 |
| 46–50 | 1.1 | 94.9 | 1.2 | 91.9 | 1.1 | 93.8 |
| 50+ | 5.1 | 100.0 | 8.0 | 99.9 | 6.1 | 99.9 |

in stoma nurse districts to have a shorter length of stay postoperatively, with one exception. This district was one which made considerable use of convalescent beds and the average length of stay for the 24 patients sampled was 34 days. In the non stoma nurse district, which also made extensive use of convalescent beds, the average length of stay was 25.4 days. This difference leads one to suppose that there might be a difference in policy towards the discharge of ostomates, and the interview with the stoma care nurse appeared to confirm this:

'We are lucky here that we have a convalescent hospital so I always insist that the majority go to convalesce, then they can really get back on their feet. Patients spend about two to two and a half weeks here and one to one and a half weeks convalescing. It varies tremendously depending on what they are going home to and how strong they are.'

It became evident, in interviews with ward sisters and stoma care nurses, that whereas there was wide agreement that a patient must be considered medically fit and able to cope with the new stoma, the time at which patients were expected to reach this point differed. For example, in some districts the policy was to discharge patients 10–14 days after surgery, yet in other districts a minimum period of 3 weeks was considered appropriate.

The majority of ward sisters and stoma care nurses who were interviewed stated that they were either consulted by surgeons with regard to the discharge of patients or could veto a decision when they felt that it was premature. For example:

'The surgeon makes the decision but asks me if the patient is ready.'

'Patients are discharged within 10–14 days, due to pressure on the surgical beds. Sometimes we just have to put our foot down and say "No, she is only 8 days".'

## Discussion

It would seem from the above data that postoperative length of stay in hospital is dependent not only on the patient's condition but also on local policy and on the current pressure on surgical beds. It seems possible that, where there is a stoma care nurse in post and pressure on surgical beds is high, patients may be discharged sooner. On the other hand, it also seems possible that the presence of a stoma care nurse, in conjunction with lower pressure on surgical beds, may lead to a longer stay in hospital.

It would seem that there is no consensus with regard to the time it takes for a patient to recover from stoma surgery and learn how to cope with a new stoma. In one district patients spent much longer in hospital/convalescent home than patients did elsewhere and this appeared to stem from the influence of the stoma care nurse. In some of the other stoma care nurse districts, where pressure on surgical beds was high, patients were discharged much sooner.

(Eighteen patients in the sample were discharged in less than 11 days and 3 patients were discharged on the seventh day following surgery.) Clearly there is a need for an evaluation of the implications of this difference in policy for the patient. Does a shorter length of stay allow sufficient time for patients to learn to cope with their new stoma and for them to be fitted with an appliance of their choice before going home? The reluctance of patients to change the type of appliance that they are used to is well known among stoma care nurses. If patients are discharged wearing a postoperative appliance are they subsequently resistant to change? Two of the stoma care nurses interviewed said that they did not find it possible to fit a patient with appliances suitable for long-term use when they were discharged 10 days following surgery.

It would appear that there is an argument for the siting of stomas to become an accepted part of the role of the stoma care nurse. The increasing interest of ward sisters in performing this task in districts without access to a stoma care nurse supports the view that this should be a nursing task. Although the majority of patients found their stoma easily visible (and therefore easier to manage), it can be argued that a figure of 1 in 7 patients who found it difficult is still too high.

The varied reactions of patients to their stoma are much more difficult to interpret. For example, one half of the sample reported positive affect. Whereas some of this may have been due to 'trade off' in terms of relief from pain or longstanding illness, it could also be attributed to denial. We could, for instance, ask how realistic it is to feel pleased following surgical mutilation. One of the stoma care nurses elaborated on this theme saying that the bereavement aspect was very relevant and that patients had to go through this. She preferred to find patients who were antagonistic initially as she believed that those who said that they were not worried or that it didn't matter could well have problems later.

In other areas of psychological testing it is commonplace for women to obtain higher scores than men, and this has been attributed to cultural values which make it more acceptable for women to express their feelings. Thus, sex differences in reported reaction to the stoma may reflect either greater negative affect on the part of females (who may be more concerned with their body image than males), a greater element of denial in the reporting of negative affect by males, or a combination of these two factors.

The finding that greater negative affect was reported by those who had had emergency surgery is easier to interpret. It would appear to underline the importance of preoperative preparation. Based on this premise one would also have expected a difference in reported affect between patients in the two sets of districts but there does not appear to be such a difference. If, however, we accept that preoperative preparation is important but that ward staff are also effective in giving this information then, when there is no stoma care nurse available, then these two findings can be reconciled. The figures from this study show a distinct improvement when compared with those from previous studies. It may, therefore, be that nurses generally are now more aware of the needs of the stoma patient than before. It is worthy of note that when asked who had been particularly helpful during their hospital stay ward nurses were cited more frequently than stoma care nurses.

In contrast, greater involvement of the family and a lower level of resistance to family involvement was found for patients in stoma nurse districts. A greater proportion of these patients also felt that they had had sufficient practice in changing their appliance before being discharged. These findings may be directly attributable to the efforts of stoma care nurses.

The value to the patient of visits by an established ostomate has been documented in previous studies. It is therefore surprising to find that the percentage of patients who received such a visit is so small.

## Summary

(1) Ninety-two per cent of stomas sited by stoma care nurses were easily visible to the patient compared with 84% of those sited by surgeons (list cases only).

(2) One third of the patients reported an extremely negative reaction on seeing their stoma for the first time. Negative affect was greater for females than for males and greater for acute admissions than for list cases.

(3) Family involvement was greater for patients in stoma nurse districts.

(4) Proportionately more patients in stoma nurse districts said that they had had sufficient practice in changing their appliance before discharge.

(5) Forty-one per cent of patients in non stoma nurse districts had received a visit from a company nurse during their stay in hospital.

(6) Only 1 in 5 patients had received a visit from an established ostomate.

(7) The average postoperative length of stay in hospital/convalescent home was 22.1 days for patients in stoma nurse districts and 24.1 days in non stoma nurse districts. There was wide variation in postoperative length of stay between districts which appeared to be related to different policies towards discharge and pressure on surgical beds.

# 6

# Returning Home

'The district and the stoma nurse
Prevented me from feeling worse.'

The first few days following discharge from hospital can be a difficult time for the person who has to adjust to life with a new stoma:

'When I first came home I was terribly nervous, I used to stand and shake in the bathroom. I felt lost.'

In the interviews, at approximately 10 weeks after surgery, patients were asked about the sources of help and support that they had received since they returned home. They were also asked about their visits to the out-patients department, the surgery and stoma clinics. Information was obtained on dietary changes, physical symptoms and readmissions to hospital. Patients were also asked for their views on self-help groups.

## Formal support

### Stoma care nurses

In stoma nurse districts 93% of patients had received at least one visit from a stoma care nurse by the time that they were interviewed. These visits were greatly appreciated by most patients:

'The stoma nurse was most helpful after I came out of hospital, she came here and she made me do it (change the appliance) in front of her in the bathroom and I got on from there.'

However, there was an occasional hitch:

'The stoma nurse and my doctor were on holiday, it was 14 days before I saw anyone, if it wasn't for the lady down the chemist . . .'

In non stoma nurse districts, 7% of patients had also seen a stoma care nurse. A minority of patients saw stoma care nurses whom they or their relatives knew about, or had met informally. However, in most cases stoma care nurses had been asked, by district nurses, to visit the patient to deal with intractable problems. For example, one very old lady whose bag had 'burst' three times in hospital and again after returning home was seen by a stoma care nurse from a neighbouring district at the request of a district nurse. Another patient who said that he had not been given any information about the supply of appliances and that he had not had any practice in changing his bag before going home because the bag had not been changed, commented about the lack of knowledge of hospital staff. He also described how, when the district nurse changed the bag, the stoma was 'full of ulcers'. At the request of the district nurse a stoma care nurse from another district came to see this patient in her spare time and, according to the patient, commented that the bag he was wearing 'went out with the ark'.

Stoma care nurses were asked about the frequency and timing of visits to patients after discharge. It appeared that the number of visits to patients over the first year following discharge varied from 1 to 10 depending on their particular policy.

The stoma care nurses in five districts said that they visited patients within the first 48 hours following discharge. The stoma care nurses in three districts said that they visited patients within the first week. In the four remaining districts, stoma care nurses said that visits were made within the first two weeks, but two nurses said that they arranged for district nurses to call within the first 48 hours following discharge.

One stoma care nurse elaborated on the importance of these visits to patients:

> 'It is a great comfort to a patient if a nurse calls—having the comfort of nurses constantly being there (in hospital) and then being totally isolated with this new thing. We always ask a district nurse to be involved, we let her know that a patient is in that area for future reasons. Many of the patients leave hospital very capable people but it is the psychological support that they need at that time.'

In 9 out of the 12 districts, the stoma care nurses had a flexible policy and visited those patients whom they felt to be at risk more frequently than others. Old people who were living alone tended to fall into this category:

> 'It is very individual, a younger patient may cope all right so you might only go and see them two or three times at home. Your elderly are always a problem, particularly if they live alone. You have to think of mobility, eyesight and dexterity and these I look at preoperatively.'

In the three districts in which stoma care nurses had a fixed policy towards home visits, one covered a very large geographical area. In another, the stoma care nurse said that she ensured that patients were independent before being discharged so that extra visits were unnecessary and that she spent more time with terminally ill patients. The third district was one in which patients tended to be discharged 10 days following surgery. These patients were visited once only and then attended a follow-up clinic 6 weeks after surgery.

All the stoma care nurses who were interviewed operated a telephone service for their patients. The number of phone calls received each week was estimated at between 10 and 20. Estimates of the proportion of patients who did call at one time or another ranged from 50 to 70%.

The majority of stoma care nurses also held clinics which patients could attend either by appointment or by simply 'dropping in' when attending the out-patient department. By the time of these first interviews one fifth of the patients in stoma nurse districts had attended one of these clinics. Five per cent of patients just 'called in', the remainder (15%) came either to consult the stoma care nurse or to obtain a further supply of appliances.

In non stoma nurse districts some of the ward sisters also held clinics which patients could attend, but less than 5% of patients had done so.

### Social workers

Eleven per cent of patients had received visits from a social worker and there was little difference between the two sets of districts. Two-thirds of the patients who had received these visits described them as helpful.

### General practitioners

By the time the patients were interviewed, 73% had been visited by their GP and two-thirds of these described the visit as helpful. Three per cent of patients said that these visits were unhelpful, and this was usually due to the fact that the doctor did not know much about stomas or stoma care appliances. Five per cent of patients said that they would have liked a visit and 22% said that they had not needed a visit.

Approximately one half of the patients had been to see their GP at the surgery. The main reasons for these visits were to obtain prescriptions (16%), to consult the doctor about some other apparently unrelated condition (12%) or to obtain a sick note (11%). A minority of patients had consulted their GP because of difficulties relating to the stoma (2%). The remaining patients had either been for a check-up (6%), for treatment or further tests (2%).

### Visits to out-patients

Two-thirds of the sample had visited the out-patients department for routine follow-up examination and a further 8.8% for tests or treatment. One in eight of the patients who had attended out-patients said that they had not found the visit very helpful. The most common complaint was that they had not been examined and that the visit was a waste of their time. For example:

'I went into a little room and he stood as far from here to there off and he said "Just lift your skirt up" and I lifted my skirt up and he said "Oh, it's all right, come back in 3 month's time". He never saw it because he couldn't see through. He never examined me, I might as well have stopped at home.'

### District nurses

Over the whole sample, 68% of patients had been visited by a district nurse. The proportion was greater for patients in non stoma nurse districts, where 82% of patients had received a visit compared with 61% of patients in stoma nurse districts. Only 3% of patients who had not seen a district nurse said that they would have liked to have seen one. Ten per cent of patients said that visits from the district nurse had not been helpful. Several of these patients, mainly in districts without stoma care nurses, reported either that the district nurse did not know anything about stomas or that they were not interested in the stoma and just came to dress the wound. Other comments related to the efforts of the district nurse to contact a stoma care nurse on behalf of the patient.

## Informal support

### Company nurses

In stoma nurse districts, 4% of patients had seen a company nurse since being discharged from hospital. Usually these patients had contacted the nurse themselves. Most patients said that these nurses were very helpful and several patients commented that they did not push their particular product.

In non stoma nurse districts, 46% of patients had been visited by a company nurse since being discharged. Most of these patients described these visits as very helpful. Only one patient said that the nurse had pushed her own product and had insisted on supplying a closed bag when the patient, an ileostomate, required a drainable appliance.

One of the ward sisters, who was interviewed later, was less approving of 'company nurses'. She had learned that patients were being charged service fees by one representative and now she debarred all company nurses/representatives from her ward. It is worth noting here that, including those who had already seen a company nurse in hospital, 61% of these patients had now seen a company nurse/representative.

### Established ostomates

Over the whole sample, only 5% of patients had been visited at home by a person with an established stoma, but a further 17% said that they would have liked a visit. Proportionately twice as many patients in non stoma nurse districts would have liked to have been able to talk to someone else who had a stoma.

## Self-help groups

We have already seen that 59% of patients said that they had not been informed of the existence of self-help groups such as the Ileostomy Association, the Colostomy Welfare Group or the Urostomy Association (Chapter 5). At 10 weeks following surgery, it is not surprising that few patients (3.8%) had actually contacted one of these organisations. However, when asked, one quarter of the sample said that they would be interested in contacting such a group. The remainder said that they were not interested, usually because they assumed either that meetings would be too far distant for them to attend or that the people attending would be commiserating with each other. Patients did not tend to view these groups as a source of positive help.

## Patient perceptions of the value of support

Patients were asked who had been the most helpful person to them since they were discharged from hospital. Their responses to this question are given, for the two sets of districts, in Table 6.1.

The value of the support and help given by a husband or wife is clearly

**Table 6.1**  Patient perceptions: those who have been of most help since discharge

|  | Stoma nurse districts (n = 176) % | Non stoma nurse districts (n = 87) % | All (n = 263) % |
| --- | --- | --- | --- |
| Spouse | 40.9 | 46.6 | 43.0 |
| Other relative | 17.6 | 15.9 | 17.1 |
| Friends/neighbours | 4.0 | 6.8 | 4.9 |
| Stoma care nurse | 19.9 | 0.0 | 13.3 |
| Company nurse | 1.1 | 8.0 | 3.4 |
| District nurse | 1.1 | 11.5 | 4.6 |
| General Practitioner | 2.3 | 4.5 | 3.0 |
| Social services staff | 2.3 | 0.0 | 1.5 |
| Patient himself | 2.8 | 2.3 | 2.7 |
| Other | 2.3 | 1.1 | 1.6 |
| No one particularly | 5.7 | 3.4 | 4.9 |
| *Total* | 100.0 | 100.1 | 100.0 |

illustrated; however the figures are misleading, for taken as a proportion of those who were married, 63% of patients said that their spouse had been the greatest source of help to them since they had come home. Other relatives were also said to have been very supportive and were cited by 17.1% of the total sample. Friends or neighbours were mentioned by a further 4.9%. For patients in stoma nurse districts the stoma care nurse figures prominently as a source of help and support and was cited by one fifth of the sample. Few of these patients mentioned the district nurse. For patients in the other districts, the district nurse or a company nurse were more frequently mentioned by patients.

A minority of patients said that other personnel, such as GPs or home helps had been of most help to them since they came home from hospital. A few patients insisted they had helped themselves and would not name anyone else.

Patients were also asked whom they would contact if they needed help with their stoma. Responses to this question are given, by type of district, in Table 6.2.

Clearly, the stoma care nurse is seen as a major source of help. More than three-quarters of the patients in stoma nurse districts said that they would contact the stoma care nurse. In the other districts, approximately one quarter of ostomates said that they would contact the district nurse and another quarter said that they would get in touch with a company nurse. The proportion of patients who said that they would contact their GP or hospital staff was also greater in this set of districts.

Approximately 10% of the whole sample said that they would contact relatives, friends or neighbours if they needed some help with their stoma. This is perhaps surprising for those patients who had access to a stoma care nurse.

**Table 6.2**   Potential source of help for stoma care, by type of district

|  | Stoma nurse districts (n = 176) % | Non stoma nurse districts (n = 87) % |
|---|---|---|
| Stoma care nurse | 77.3 | 1.1 |
| Company nurse | 1.1 | 25.3 |
| District nurse | 2.3 | 27.6 |
| General practitioner | 7.4 | 18.4 |
| Hospital staff | 0.6 | 12.6 |
| Relatives/friends/neighbours | 10.8 | 10.3 |
| Established ostomate | 0.0 | 2.3 |
| Other | 0.6 | 0.0 |
| Don't know | 0.0 | 2.3 |
| *Total* | 100.1 | 99.9 |

## Modifications to diet

Patients were asked if they had changed their diet in any way since they had had surgery and, if so, whether these changes were made as a consequence of surgery. Over the whole sample 76.4% of ostomates had modified their diet and 68.8% attributed the change to having a stoma. Almost two-thirds of those who had changed their diet had restricted it by at least one item of food whereas the remainder said that they now ate some foods that they didn't eat before. The pattern of dietary change was very similar for patients in the two sets of districts. Fewer dietary changes had been made by patients with urinary stomas.

The biggest single change was in the consumption of vegetables. Whereas

**Table 6.3**  Percentage of patients adding or excluding items from their diet

|  | Items eliminated (n = 263) % | Items added (n = 263) % |
|---|---|---|
| All vegetables | 2.7 | 3.0 |
| Onions | 21.7 | 0.0 |
| Peas/beans | 14.0 | 0.4 |
| Greens/salad | 11.0 | 1.5 |
| Tomatoes | 4.2 | 0.4 |
| Root vegetables | 3.0 | 0.4 |
| Other vegetables | 1.2 | 0.0 |
| All fruit | 6.8 | 5.7 |
| Citrus fruit | 4.6 | 2.3 |
| Fruit with seeds/pips | 5.3 | 0.4 |
| Dried fruit | 1.9 | 0.8 |
| Bananas | 1.1 | 0.4 |
| Other fruit | 1.5 | 1.1 |
| Nuts | 8.7 | 0.0 |
| All meat | 1.1 | 0.0 |
| Red meat | 1.9 | 0.8 |
| Processed meats | 1.9 | 0.4 |
| Chicken | 0.0 | 0.4 |
| Bran | 0.8 | 8.0 |
| Bran products | 1.1 | 3.8 |
| Wholemeal/brown bread | 1.1 | 3.0 |
| Cereals | 1.5 | 3.8 |
| Cakes/pastries/sweets | 5.3 | 2.3 |
| Curries/spiced foods | 8.4 | 0.8 |
| Dairy products | 3.0 | 3.4 |
| Fish | 0.8 | 0.8 |
| Dried foods | 3.4 | 0.0 |
| Other foods | 1.9 | 1.1 |
| Alcoholic drinks | 2.7 | 0.8 |
| Fruit juice | 1.5 | 1.1 |

6.1% of patients were now eating more vegetables than before, 57.8% of patients had eliminated at least one vegetable from their diet (Table 6.3). Onions, peas/beans and green vegetables were the items most commonly eliminated.

There was also a considerable change in the consumption of fruit: 21.3% of the sample had reduced their consumption by at least one item, but exactly half as many patients (10.6%) now ate items of fruit that they did not eat before they had surgery. Nuts were no longer eaten by 8.7% of patients, and curries or highly spiced foods had now been eliminated from their diet by 8.4% of patients. A small proportion of patients had reduced their consumption of meat (4.9%) and others had reduced their consumption of sweet foods (5.3%). The biggest single addition to the diet was of bran or bran products (11.8%).

Similar findings to those reported here have been found in previous research (Gazzard and Dawson, 1978). It is suggested that rigid dietary instruction would be inappropriate because patients react differently to various foods (Elcoat, 1986).

## Physical symptoms

Complete recovery from major surgery could hardly be expected after only 10 weeks and this was confirmed by patients' responses to the items on the physical symptoms scale (PSS). For example, more than one half of the whole sample had experienced some pain since returning home from hospital and one quarter of the sample described this as very or extremely severe. At the time of the interview more than one third of the sample said that they still had pain and 8.7% described it as very or extremely severe like the following male patient who had a permanent colostomy:

'I knew I was going to experience some discomfort but it was very severe, dreadful, I must admit that I shed a tear, in private.'

The percentage of patients who had experienced different symptoms and who still had symptoms are given in Table 6.4. It can be seen that fatigue was still a problem at the time of these first interviews, three-quarters of the sample experienced tiredness to some degree and extreme fatigue was reported by more than one in ten patients. One third of the patients said that they had backache; this was more common among ileostomates of whom one quarter described it as severe.

One fifth of the patients reported indigestion but only 4% described it as severe or very frequent. Nausea and vomiting were less frequent overall but were slightly more common among ileostomates. One in 10 patients said that they were constipated to some extent, but this particular problem was much more common among urostomates. Diarrhoea was a more common com-

**Table 6.4**  Physical symptoms experienced by patients (a) since discharge from hospital and (b) at 10 weeks postoperatively

| | Symptoms experienced since discharge (n = 263) | | Symptoms at time of interview (n = 263) | |
|---|---|---|---|---|
| | *To some extent* % | *Often or severe* % | *To some extent* % | *Often or severe* % |
| Fatigue | 89.7 | 70.0 | 74.1 | 12.9 |
| Pain | 51.7 | 29.8 | 39.9 | 8.7 |
| Backache | 38.4 | 12.9 | 34.6 | 8.7 |
| Sweating | 19.8 | 5.7 | 17.9 | 4.6 |
| Indigestion | 20.5 | 6.5 | 18.3 | 4.2 |
| Nausea | 14.4 | 4.6 | 8.7 | 1.1 |
| Vomiting | 12.5 | 4.9 | 4.6 | 0.8 |
| Constipation | 17.1 | 6.5 | 10.3 | 2.3 |
| Diarrhoea | 31.2 | 12.9 | 21.7 | 6.1 |
| Incontinence (urine)[1] | 7.8 | 3.7 | 6.2 | 0.8 |
| Urinary infection | 11.8 | 5.3 | 4.9 | 1.1 |
| Abdominal wound infection | 16.0 | 7.0 | 4.9 | 1.6 |
| Perineal wound infection[2] | 44.5 | 29.7 | 26.5 | 3.9 |
| Discharge (other) | 24.7 | 10.6 | 19.8 | 4.6 |
| Prolapse of stoma | 2.7 | 0.8 | 4.2 | 0.4 |
| Retraction of stoma | 3.8 | 0.8 | 7.6 | 1.1 |
| Stenosis of stoma | 0.4 | 0.4 | 1.1 | 0.0 |
| Hernia of stoma | 2.3 | 1.1 | 2.3 | 1.5 |
| Obstruction of stoma | 3.4 | 3.0 | 0.8 | 0.0 |
| Slight bleeding of stoma | 63.9 | 3.4 | 46.4 | 1.9 |
| Severe bleeding of stoma | 3.0 | 1.1 | 1.9 | 0.4 |
| Ulcers of stoma | 3.4 | 1.5 | 3.0 | 0.4 |
| Infection of stoma | 3.0 | 1.9 | 1.5 | 0.0 |
| Flatus[1] | 82.3 | 35.4 | 80.2 | 23.0 |
| Smell | 56.7 | 11.9 | 47.7 | 7.4 |
| Noise[1] | 73.7 | 10.7 | 70.4 | 6.2 |
| Sensation of rectal fullness[2] | 67.9 | 17.2 | 72.7 | 8.6 |

[1] Bowel stomas only (n = 243)
[2] Permanent bowel stomas only (n = 136)

plaint, and this occurred twice as frequently in ileostomates, of whom one fifth described it as severe.

Urinary infections, though infrequent, were not confined to those patients with urinary stomas. Six per cent of patients with bowel stomas said that they had some degree of incontinence of urine.

The abdominal wound had healed for most patients but one quarter of those who had had abdominoperineal excision of the rectum said that their perineum had not fully healed or was painful.

Slight bleeding of the stoma, which is often associated with over zealous cleaning, was quite common, but severe bleeding was rare. Ulcers, or infections of the stoma itself were also rarely reported.

The majority of patients with bowel stomas said that they suffered from flatus, and almost one quarter said that this affected them frequently. This symptom was more common among ileostomates of whom more than one third said that it happened often. Similarly, a greater proportion of ileostomates said that their stoma was noisy. On the other hand, a greater proportion of colostomates said that there was some degree of smell associated with the stoma. Overall, 7.4% of patients said that they often or very often noticed the smell, and this particular item gave rise to far more spontaneous comments than any other. For example:

'I have a horror of the thought that I might smell.'

'There is nothing worse that to sit and have an odour coming from you, I should die a thousand deaths. I quietly take this out of my pocket and spray it and put it back. This is what I am doing all the time, I'd be a bag of nerves if I didn't. If only they'd make a bag that the filter would definitely work.'

'They all say they can't smell—I do—I wear disinfectant, I think they don't like to tell me.'

'The smell permeates the whole house, I have to open doors and windows and everything. Two to three weeks ago my wife said "Oh God—for God's sake!" she has the front door open, the back door and she was right, it was really awful.'

'I can smile through pain and nobody need know; I can live with it but the smell with the new bags is embarassing, undignified and I feel very strongly about it.'

'When I empty my bag the stink is dreadful, it goes through the whole house and I have to empty this at least 6 times a day. It's like a creeping lurgy, it is insidious.'

Clearly some patients appeared to be unduly worried that they might smell, despite reassurances that they did not. Others accepted such reassurances. However, there is no doubt that, for a minority of patients, odour really was a problem which often arose when changing, or draining the bag. Moreover, it appeared, on interview, that many of the patients who complained about smell were wearing drainable bags.

According to Devlin (1976a), up to 40% of patients experience feelings of tenesmus and curious sensations which have been labelled 'phantom rectum'. At the time of the interviews, almost three-quarters of those patients who had a permanent bowel stoma reported that they were still experiencing a sensation of rectal fullness, although less than 1 in 10 patients said that they often or very often had this feeling. However, many of the temporary ostomates whose rectum was preserved, also reported this sensation. In some, but not all, cases this appeared to be due to the accumulation of mucus or faecal residue. It seems possible that the attribution of the phenomenon of the 'phantom rectum' to psychological rather than physiological disturbance may not always be justified.

Devlin (1976b) describes 5 structural complications of colostomy; stenosis, retraction, prolapse, obstruction and herniation adjacent to the stoma. Stenosis, as a complication of colostomy, is unusual (Abrams, 1984). As a complication of ileostomy, stenosis is extremely rare since the advent of the eversion ileostomy described by Brooke in 1952 (Walker, 1976). Stenosis of the ileal conduit can occur due to strictures or constriction where the conduit passes through the abdominal wall (Elcoat, 1986). Retraction of the stoma, like prolapse, may be due to inadequate fixing of the stoma but can also occur with postoperative gain in weight. Obstruction may occur due to adhesions, volvulus or a bolus of undigested fruit or vegetables. Herniation is a complication which occurs more frequently in colostomates than in ileostomates, but pseudohernia, due to placement of the stoma lateral to the rectus muscle which may stretch over time giving rise to a bulge, can also occur (Kretschmer, 1978).

During these first interviews, 4% of patients described some degree of prolapse, but only one patient who had a 'temporary' colostomy said that this was severe. Some retraction of the stoma was described by 7.6% of patients, but severe retraction was described by two patients with permanent colostomies and one patient with a 'temporary' colostomy. Stenosis of the stoma was rare, two colostomates and one urostomate described a slight stenosis. Almost 3% of colostomates said that they thought they had a hernia and four patients whose stomas were 'temporary' described it as severe. Some degree of obstruction had been experienced by 3.4% of patients but, as indicated in the next section, only one patient had been readmitted for this particular reason.

Although these structural complications may be more serious from a surgical standpoint, there is little doubt that the problems that were uppermost in the minds of many patients were related to stoma management and the possibility of smell.

## Readmissions

At approximately 10 weeks following surgery, 30 patients (11.4%) had either been readmitted to hospital (9.5%) or were about to be readmitted for reasons other than reversal of stoma. The reasons for readmission are given in Table 6.5.

The complications described by patients included muscle spasm, obstruction, abscess and bladder damage. Two patients were readmitted because the formal support system had broken down. Both of these readmissions were in non stoma nurse districts. One patient could not fix his own appliance due to physical problems, and his wife had not been told how to care for him. He was discharged at the weekend and no district nurse was available. He was readmitted for 3 days. The second patient, an ex-nurse who was very ill, was

**Table 6.5**   Ten weeks after surgery: reasons
for readmission

| Reasons for readmission | Number |
| --- | --- |
| Other apparently unrelated conditions | 8 |
| Complications | 6 |
| Resiting/refashioning of stoma | 3 |
| Second stage surgery | 2 |
| Drain removal | 2 |
| Pain treatment/chemotherapy | 2 |
| Depression/anxiety | 2 |
| Reversal (not done) | 1 |
| Ileostomy (colostomate) | 1 |
| Social reasons | 1 |
| Lack of formal support | 2 |
| *Total* | 30 |

discharged having been assured that she would be cared for by the district nursing service. However she reported that:

'We had four district nurses in this room all saying "Well we just don't know what to do'! They knew nothing, they had no equipment and no knowledge.'

The GP tried, in vain, to locate a stoma care nurse but the patient had to be readmitted.

## Discussion

It is apparent that discharge policy varied across the districts. It would seem that stoma care nurses also differ in their policy with regard to home visits. For, although most patients in stoma nurse districts were visited within the first week of discharge, the number of subsequent visits varied and could be affected by the size of the district or by according a higher priority to the care of terminally ill ostomates. Despite these differences, most stoma care nurses said that their policy was flexible and that they tended to visit some patients, usually the elderly who were living alone, more frequently than others.

Company nurses/representatives featured quite prominently in non stoma nurse districts. At 10 weeks following surgery, two-thirds of the patients in these districts had seen a company nurse at some point but, whereas more than three-quarters of patients in stoma nurse districts named the stoma care nurse as the person they would contact if they had problems with their stoma, only one quarter of patients in other districts said that they would get in touch with a company nurse. Indeed, patients were just as likely to mention the district nurse. Judging by the variety of people named, it would seem that patients in these districts do not see any one person as a major source of potential help.

The physical symptoms which patients reported at 10 weeks following surgery give some cause for concern. For example, in addition to problems arising from the stoma, the proportion of patients who were still suffering, to some extent, from fatigue, pain, backache, gastrointestinal upset or wound problems was considerable. Yet, as will be shown in the next chapter, despite these problems the majority of patients were independent with regard to the management of appliances.

## Summary

At 10 weeks following surgery:

(1) The majority of patients in stoma nurse districts were visited within 1 week of being discharged.

(2) One in 8 patients spontaneously said that their visit to the out-patients department was unhelpful or a waste of time.

(3) Two-thirds of the sample had been visited by a district nurse, the proportion being greater in non stoma nurse districts where patients were more likely to say that district nurses knew nothing about stoma care.

(4) Almost one half of patients in non stoma nurse districts had been visited at home by a company nurse/representative. Sixty-one per cent of patients in non stoma nurse districts had seen a company nurse/representative at some point since surgery.

(5) Only 5% of patients had been visited at home by an established ostomate, but a further 17% said that they would have liked a visit (the proportion being much greater in non stoma nurse districts).

(6) One quarter of the sample said that they would be interested in joining a self-help group.

(7) The stoma care nurse is seen as the major source of help in stoma nurse districts. A variety of people was named by patients in other districts.

(8) Three-quarters of patients had modified their diet, mainly by restricting at least one item of food.

(9) The most frequently reported symptoms were fatigue, pain, backache, diarrhoea and, for those patients with bowel stomas, a sensation of rectal fullness, flatus, noise, odour and problems with the perineal wound.

(10) Of the sample, 11.4% had either been readmitted to hospital or were about to be readmitted for reasons other than reversal of stoma.

# 7

# Appliances: Management and Satisfaction

'What's that projecting from my tum,
All pink and wrinkled like a plum?
It's what we call a stoma, mate,
You use it as an exit gate.'

A considerable part of these first interviews with patients was devoted to the management of appliances. Patients were asked whether they had had any difficulty in obtaining their supply of appliances, what type of appliance they used and whether they managed to change the appliance by themselves. They were also asked if they had changed to a different type of bag since they had come home from hospital and whether they had made any modifications to their current appliance to make it more suitable for them. Finally, their satisfaction with the appliance was assessed using the scales described in Chapter 2.

## Obtaining appliances

Over the whole sample, 36 patients (13.7%) said that they had had difficulties in obtaining their supply of equipment. The most common problem lay in establishing their supply after being discharged from hospital (6.5%). Some patients had had to wait 3 weeks before their order at the chemist was completed. The need to make at least two visits to the chemist was a problem for some patients who had to travel a considerable distance from their home. Other patients had prescription difficulties (3.4%). Either their own doctor was on holiday or had not been informed about the patient or the wrong size, type or quantity of appliances was prescribed. Problems with the chemist were infrequent (2.3%) but could be distressing. For example, one chemist refused to obtain a supply and two others argued with patients over the cost of appliances:

'He said "You cannot possibly use all these bags, they are £40 a box!"'

## Types of appliance in use

Patients were asked which make of appliance they used and these were inspected to find out whether the bag was drainable or closed, whether it was a 1-piece appliance, used with or without a wafer, or a 2-piece appliance (defined for this purpose as one which has a separate flange). Although 9 brands of appliance were identified 3 brands were used by 88% of the total sample. Four patients (1.5%) were using 2 different brands.

Postoperatively, it is usual for patients to be fitted with a drainable appliance made of transparent material which allows observation of the stoma. However, at 10 weeks following surgery one would expect that postoperative oedema of the stoma would have subsided and that patients would be wearing an appliance which is suitable to their life-style and appropriate to their stoma. It will be recalled that almost three-quarters of the sample said that their stoma had changed shape and that the majority of these also said that it was now smaller. It has already been noted (Chapter 4) that far more of the patients in stoma nurse districts recalled being told about the different types of appliance available, when compared with patients in non stoma nurse districts. Is there any evidence to suggest that some patients may have been using an inappropriate appliance?

Analysis of the data revealed that 34.1% of permanent colostomates in non stoma nurse districts were still using a drainable appliance compared with 15.9% of their counterparts in stoma nurse districts. This difference between the two sets of patients is statistically significant ($\chi^2$ 1 d.f. = 4.68, $P < 0.05$). Whereas a drainable bag may be appropriate for some permanent colostomates and others may actually prefer it, one would not expect the difference in proportions between the two sets of districts to be so large. Moreover, some patients who were equipped with drainable bags did not use them as such, preferring to change the bag 'because of the odour'. In contrast, a greater proportion of 'temporary' colostomates in stoma nurse districts (31.5%) were using a drainable appliance than their counterparts in non stoma nurse districts (25%). This difference is not statistically significant. The number of ileostomates is rather small but one would expect that all these patients would be wearing a drainable appliance. The 17 ileostomates in stoma nurse districts were indeed using a drainable appliance but 2 of the 11 ileostomates in non stoma nurse districts (one of whom had been seen by a company nurse) were using closed bags and a further patient, who had also been seen by a company nurse, volunteered that 'she tended to push her own product' and argued with him when he told her that he needed a drainable appliance. The patient now has a box of closed bags which he cannot use.

In one non stoma nurse district, most of the patients interviewed were wearing inappropriate appliances. For example, one woman with a permanent colostomy who, before surgery, used to wear tights and little cotton briefs could no longer do so. She was wearing a very long drainable bag and had had to purchase long-legged knickers to accommodate this. She also produced what she thought were plastic covers for the bag but which were in fact disposal bags. In trying to adjust to life with a stoma, this woman was keen to learn and had read five books on stoma care. She found these unsatisfactory for several reasons. One of the books stated that you could train the stoma to work at a regular time and she questioned the possibility of this. She also questioned the possibility of swimming which she enjoyed.

'I cannot imagine how—I mean I couldn't go swimming. I couldn't conceal this thing under a swimming suit.'

Over the whole sample 53% of patients were using a one-piece appliance, a further 10% were using a one-piece appliance, together with a wafer, and 37% of patients were using a two-piece appliance. There was little difference in these proportions between the two sets of districts.

## Changes in the type of appliance used

Thirty-six patients in stoma nurse districts (20.5%) and 26 patients in non stoma nurse districts (29.9%) had changed to a different appliance since leaving hospital. The reasons given for these changes are listed in Table 7.1 for the two sets of districts. For the most part, the reasons given are those of simple preference but 10 patients, who had changed to a different type of

**Table 7.1**  Reasons given for change in type of appliance since discharge from hospital, by type of district

| Reasons for change | Stoma nurse districts (n = 176) % | Non stoma nurse districts (n = 87) % | All (n = 263) % |
|---|---|---|---|
| Preferred a drainable bag | 0.0 | 3.5 | 1.1 |
| Preferred a sealed bag | 1.1 | 5.7 | 2.7 |
| Preferred a 1-piece bag | 1.7 | 3.5 | 2.3 |
| Preferred a 2-piece bag | 1.1 | 0.0 | 0.8 |
| Preferred a bag with a filter | 2.3 | 1.1 | 1.9 |
| Management difficulties | 0.6 | 1.1 | 0.8 |
| Leakage | 2.8 | 4.6 | 3.4 |
| Skin sensitivity | 2.8 | 1.1 | 2.3 |
| Discomfort | 1.7 | 0.0 | 1.1 |
| Lacked confidence | 1.1 | 2.3 | 1.5 |
| Other reasons, e.g. size, shape | 4.5 | 5.7 | 4.9 |
| Difficulty in obtaining appliance | 0.6 | 1.1 | 0.8 |
| No change | 79.5 | 70.1 | 76.4 |
| *Total* | 99.8 | 99.8 | 100.0 |

appliance, did so because they had problems with leakage and 6 other patients said that they had changed because of skin sensitivity. When asked who had recommended the change in appliance the majority of patients in stoma nurse districts said that the stoma care nurse had done so. In other districts, company nurses had recommended the change in more than one third of cases. However, community nurses, established ostomates, general practitioners, relatives, stoma care nurses from other districts and pharmacists were also named.

### Modifications to appliances

Patients were also asked if they had modified the appliance they were using to make it more suitable for them. Just over one quarter of the sample described some form of modification that they had made (Table 7.2). The most common modification was that of trimming some part of the appliance, such as the edge of the adhesive or flange or an unwanted belt attachment. Five per cent of ostomates had modified the way in which they wore their appliance. For example, by wearing a drainable bag at an angle the clip is situated on the outside of the leg where it is less likely to cause discomfort. Another modification, which patients said prevented 'pancaking' or collapse of the bag, was to tuck the bottom of the bag up inside itself. Some patients folded up the bottom of the bag to make it shorter and two patients wore the bag outside their clothing for comfort. One man had sewn a pocket inside his underpants. This served a dual purpose since it avoided skin contact and supported the weight.

Apart from the deodorant drops which some patients used, paper tissue or talcum powder were also put into the bag to prevent 'pancaking'.

**Table 7.2**   Modifications to appliance, by type of district

| Modification | Stoma nurse districts | | Non stoma nurse districts | | All | |
|---|---|---|---|---|---|---|
| | n | % | n | % | n | % |
| Trims part of appliance | 22 | 12.5 | 5 | 5.7 | 27 | 10.3 |
| Additions | 6 | 3.4 | 5 | 5.7 | 11 | 4.2 |
| Mode of wear | 5 | 2.8 | 9 | 10.3 | 14 | 5.3 |
| Adaptations to clothing | 0 | 0.0 | 2 | 2.3 | 2 | 0.8 |
| Alters fastening mechanism | 2 | 1.1 | 2 | 2.3 | 4 | 1.5 |
| Pin holes | 6 | 3.4 | 1 | 1.1 | 7 | 2.6 |
| Home-made punch | 1 | 0.6 | 1 | 1.1 | 2 | 0.8 |
| Drainage system | 1 | 0.6 | 0 | 0.0 | 1 | 0.4 |
| Modification to filter | 1 | 0.6 | 0 | 0.0 | 1 | 0.4 |
| No modification | 132 | 75.0 | 62 | 71.3 | 194 | 73.8 |
| *Total* | 176 | 100.0 | 87 | 99.8 | 263 | 100.1 |

Seven patients said that they made pinholes in the bag to allow the escape of flatus. However, this is probably an underestimate of the number of patients who did this as sometimes they had been instructed to do so. The holes that patients made could be sealed with sticking plaster or micropore tape but one patient used chewing gum!

Three patients were more inventive. Two had made their own punch so that they could cut the wafer to the exact size and shape of their stoma and one urostomate had devised his own night drainage system.

Clips could be difficult for arthritic fingers but they could also be uncomfortable so four patients had devised a different method of closure for their drainable bags.

## Problems with appliances

Apart from the fear of smell there were two major problems which often came up in conversation with patients. The first of these was the inflation of the bag due to flatus:

'You see when you get the wind the bag lifts, and if you're out . . . this morning it seemed to be out like this. People might not have noticed it but I did. That bothers me.'

'That bag goes full of air and it's out here—my grandson said "You'd think you was expecting, grandmother".'

'My main problem is this confounded wind of a night time. I always empty the bag before we go to bed but by half past one in the morning I have to get out and get rid of this wind.'

The second major problem, described by patients, was 'pancaking' in which the sides of the bag stick together and faecal matter cannot fall down the bag:

'I tried putting bits of paper inside to stop it sticking but that doesn't work for long. If you put a bit of talcum powder in that stops it.'

'It really sticks you know, really goes flat and I have to keep trying and pulling it a bit.'

It is apparent that an inflated bag is a potential source of embarrassment to patients, but both 'blowing up. and 'pancaking' could lead to leakage or worse. In theory, one would expect that a filter, which allows the passage of air, would prevent both these problems but many patients were sceptical:

'The filter doesn't work—it still blows up.'

'I still have to stick pins into the bag.'

'It blows up when I have a filter on. Now when I haven't it sticks.'

'The filter tends to get clogged, they should put it up in a corner.'

With some filters, patients are instructed to make pin holes from the outside.

Two patients said that the filter was more effective if pricked from the inside. Some patients also criticised filters saying that they were ineffective in removing odour or that they were effective but only for a short time, or that they squeaked!

The problem of the 'pancaking' appliance was discussed with stoma care nurses:

> 'I haven't found a single filter that really works effectively. The filter alters the pressure within the bag and, depending on the amount of faeces, the filter blocks with moisture—it doesn't need to be faeces that causes the filter to block. It is mainly the bags with an integral filter that can collapse.'

> 'The bag pancakes, the faeces don't go down—it squashes out at the side causing leakage and forces the bag off.'

Disasters, in which the bag became completely detached, spilling the contents, were not rare and happened in a variety of circumstances:

> 'I was in the supermarket a fortnight ago and I was being served at the butcher's counter and it ran all down my legs. Walking from the supermarket to the car, driving home—by the time you've done all that it is everywhere. Now I am beginning to get apprehensive about going out.'

> 'I was sitting here reading one afternoon and I knew it had been working and I stood up and the whole thing came out at the side. A terrible mess.'

> 'It blew off in bed. I was so embarrassed, it made a hell of a mess. I mean I'd never done anything like that in my life and I was so embarrassed. I felt like a baby. Then damn it, the next night it almost happened again.' (This patient is now on sedatives.)

> 'Now twice I've had it seeping underneath the wafer and once it burst here because it blew up like a balloon. We go out for a drink somewhere and I'm having to go to the toilet to keep relieving the bag. At my sisters I used a pin—I didn't feel it but it went straight into my stoma, it bled like a tap. I was worried stiff.'

> 'I've had one or two accidents with the thing coming off and I got very depressed over it, upset about it. I just haven't got the confidence in the bag. I'm afraid something will happen when I'm out. It could happen anywhere at anytime in whatever company I was in. I'm still very nervous about it.'

Twenty patients described at least one such major accident with their appliance. Proportionately more of these patients were from non stoma nurse districts (12.6%) than from stoma nurse districts (5.1%). This difference is statistically significant ($\chi^2$ 1 d.f. = 4.73, $P < 0.05$).

## Self-care: changing the appliance

Over the whole sample, 82.5% of patients were able to change their appliance unaided; a further 9.1% had help and 8.4% were dependent on another person to change the appliance for them. As shown in Figure 7.1 there are differences

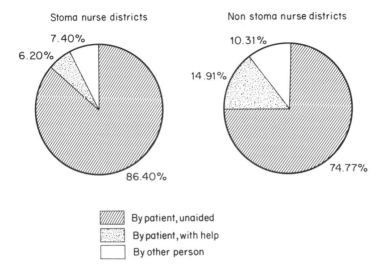

Stoma nurse districts    Non stoma nurse districts

7.40%    10.31%

6.20%

14.91%

86.40%    74.77%

By patient, unaided
By patient, with help
By other person

**Figure 7.1** Independence/dependence in changing the appliance

between the two sets of districts. In non stoma nurse districts a slightly greater proportion of patients were totally dependent on another person and more than twice as many patients had help in changing their appliance. These differences are also statistically significant ($\chi^2$ 2 d.f. = 6.46, $P < 0.05$).

The reasons why patients had help from, or were dependent on, another person are given in Table 7.3 for the two sets of districts. In some cases the position of the stoma made changing the bag very difficult, often because it was situated too high. Some patients were too ill, or too weak, had problems with their hands due to Parkinsons disease or stroke, or had poor sight. Others either needed help to apply the bag or flange firmly and in the correct position

**Table 7.3** Reasons why patients required help in changing the appliance; by type of district

| Reason why help required | Stoma nurse districts | | Non stoma nurse districts | | All | |
|---|---|---|---|---|---|---|
| | n | % | n | % | n | % |
| Position of stoma | 3 | 1.7 | 5 | 5.7 | 8 | 3.0 |
| Disablement | 9 | 5.1 | 5 | 5.7 | 14 | 5.3 |
| Difficulties in application/reassurance | 7 | 4.0 | 7 | 8.1 | 14 | 5.3 |
| Preference/staff | 4 | 2.3 | 5 | 5.7 | 9 | 3.4 |
| Depression | 1 | 0.6 | 0 | 0.0 | 1 | 0.4 |
| No help needed | 152 | 86.4 | 65 | 74.7 | 217 | 82.5 |
| *Total* | | 100.1 | | 99.9 | | 99.9 |

or felt the need for reassurance when doing this. A few patients preferred that their spouse changed the bag and sometimes the spouse preferred to do this. Staff in residential care also performed this task. The district nurse was involved in changing the appliance for two patients in non stoma nurse districts.

## Satisfaction with appliance

Appliance satisfaction was assessed in two ways. The appliance problems scale (APS) is essentially a measure of objective satisfaction inasmuch as the items relate to specific criteria such as whether the appliance leaks, gets in the way when the patient changes position, or causes skin irritation. A higher score on this scale indicates more problems. The satisfaction with appliance scale (SAS) is more a measure of subjective satisfaction, concerned with comfort, ease of fixing, confidence and overall satisfaction. A higher score on this scale indicates greater satisfaction. A Pearson product moment correlation of $-0.44$ was found between scores on these two measures at 10 weeks following surgery. These two measures are described more fully in Chapter 2.

Analysis of covariance was the method chosen to assess patient outcome based on these two measures. This is also described in Chapter 2.

The appliance problems scale (APS)

The mean score on this scale for the whole sample was 8.25 (s.d. = 2.1). The results of analysis of covariance of scores on the APS are given in Table 7.4. It is apparent that both age and physical symptoms are strongly related to

**Table 7.4**   Analysis of covariance: appliance problems

| Source of variance | Sum of squares | d.f. | Mean square | F |
|---|---|---|---|---|
| *Covariates* | | | | |
| Physical state (SQRT) | 132.662 | 1 | 132.662 | 36.346*** |
| Age | 40.913 | 1 | 40.913 | 11.209*** |
| *Main effects* | | | | |
| Type of stoma | 42.095 | 3 | 14.032 | 3.844** |
| Access to a stoma nurse | 1.740 | 1 | 1.740 | 0.477 |
| *Error* | 930.870 | 255 | 3.650 | |

*** $P < 0.001$.
 ** $P < 0.01$.
  * $P < 0.05$.

problems with appliances. After these effects have been partialled out, the extent to which patients experience problems with their appliance is significantly related to the type of stoma that they have but is unrelated to the type of district. In other words, when the scores are adjusted for age, patients who had higher scores on the physical symptoms scale also reported more problems with their appliance. On the other hand, age is negatively related to scores on the APS—having controlled for scores on the physical symptoms scale, older patients reported fewer problems with their appliance.

After controlling for the effects of age and physical symptoms, there are no significant differences in scores on the APS between patients who had access to a stoma care nurse and those who did not. There are differences in scores between patients who had different types of stoma. Those who had permanent colostomies tended to have fewer problems with their appliances than patients who had temporary colostomies or ileostomies. Patients who had urinary stomas tended to have more problems.

## The satisfaction with appliance scale (SAS)

The results of analysis of covariance of scores on the SAS are given in Table 7.5. The results of this analysis indicate that subjective satisfaction is also strongly related to physical symptoms; when the scores are adjusted for differences in age, higher scores on the physical symptoms scale are associated with lower scores on the SAS. However, when scores on the SAS are adjusted for differences in physical symptoms, age is unrelated to subjective satisfaction with appliances.

The mean (average) score on the SAS for the whole sample is 306 (s.d. = 58.6). When SAS scores are adjusted to take account of physical

**Table 7.5**  Analysis of covariance: appliance satisfaction

| Source of variance | Sum of squares | d.f. | Mean square | F |
|---|---|---|---|---|
| *Covariates* | | | | |
| Physical state (SQRT) | 90 802.282 | 1 | 90 802.282 | 29.976*** |
| Age | 1 182.065 | 1 | 1 182.065 | 0.390 |
| *Main effects* | | | | |
| Type of stoma | 9 763.084 | 3 | 3 254.361 | 1.074 |
| Access to a stoma nurse | 14 959.937 | 1 | 14 959.937 | 4.939* |
| *Error* | 772 424.744 | 255 | 3 029.117 | |

*** $P < 0.001$.
 ** $P < 0.01$.
  * $P < 0.05$.

symptoms and age, they are unrelated to the type of stoma that a patient has but they are significantly related to the type of district. In stoma nurse districts the adjusted mean score is 311 and in non stoma nurse districts it is 295. It is apparent that subjective satisfaction with appliances is greater for patients in stoma nurse districts. A separate analysis showed that patients who had had accidents in which the bag became detached had lower satisfaction (mean score 276).

It will be recalled that many of the stoma care nurses said that they placed a higher priority on the care of the elderly living alone. The mean SAS score for widowed ostomates in the upper third of the age distribution in stoma nurse districts is 320. The mean SAS score for their counterparts in non stoma nurse districts is 284. Widowed elderly ostomates in stoma nurse districts also had slightly lower scores on the appliance problems scale.

These analyses appear to indicate that the physical state of the patient, defined in terms of the number and severity of physical symptoms, is strongly related both to the extent and severity of specific problems with appliances and to subjective satisfaction with appliances. Older patients tend to report a lower incidence and severity of problems but age is, overall, unrelated to subjective satisfaction. The type of stoma that a patient has is also related to the extent and severity of problems with appliances but is unrelated to subjective satisfaction. On the other hand, access to a stoma care nurse is unrelated to specific problems but is related to subjective satisfaction with appliances.

## Discussion

In this chapter, it has been shown that appliance management, for the patient with a newly created stoma, can be fraught with problems. More than 1 in 10 patients had difficulties in establishing their supply of equipment. It is perhaps worth considering what this entails on the part of the patient. For example, in the last chapter it was stated that one half of the sample had been to see their GP and the main reason for these visits was to obtain a prescription. The necessity to place their order for equipment in advance often meant that the patient then had to make two visits to the chemist. Some of these problems could be avoided if stoma care nurses were authorised to prescribe stoma care appliances.

Some patients appeared to be using an inappropriate appliance. Since leaving hospital, approximately one quarter of the sample had changed to a different type of appliance and a similar number had either modified their appliance, or their use of the appliance, in some way.

Kretschmer (1978), says that nothing is more dreaded by a patient than unexpected spillage:

'If it occurs it produces such a profound feeling of shame and degradation that it can totally destroy progress that had been made toward rehabilitation.' (p. 117)

Similarly, Sutherland et al (1952) suggest that such events can result in depression which may be 'frankly suicidal' and that, once a spillage has occurred, the possibility that it could happen again is a constant source of anxiety. Disasters, in which the appliance became detached and caused spilling of the contents, were described less frequently in stoma nurse districts. It is also evident that a greater proportion of patients in stoma nurse districts were independent in self-care.

On the other hand, whereas the scale, devised to assess the extent of problems with appliances, did reflect differences between patients with different types of stoma it did not reveal differences between patients in stoma nurse districts and patients elsewhere. It is important to consider this finding in a wider context. For example, it will be recalled that two-thirds of ostomates in non stoma nurse districts had seen either a company nurse or a stoma care nurse from another district. There is, therefore, a considerable degree of contamination of these data. A second consideration relates to possible deficiencies in the scale used to assess appliance problems (APS). This is a brief, 5-item scale which was devised for use across all types of stoma. This decision precluded the use of items such as the collapse or inflation of bags, which would not have been relevant to urostomates. This scale is, therefore, limited in its usefulness to detect differences in the extent and severity of problems.

We have seen that some patients in non stoma nurse districts appeared to be wearing inappropriate appliances. These may not have given rise to problems, but they could affect patient satisfaction and this was greater in stoma nurse districts. This finding complements the earlier one which showed that satisfaction with information was also greater for patients in stoma nurse districts. One interpretation of these results is that it is the continuity of care provided by stoma care nurses that gives rise to greater confidence and satisfaction. This aspect of care may be missing when we consider the contribution that company nurses make, as evidenced by the finding that, whereas the stoma care nurse is seen as a major source of help by patients who had access to such a nurse, a greater variety of people was named by patients in other districts (Chapter 6).

A further major finding is the extent to which patients' perceptions of their physical state are related to both objective and subjective satisfaction with appliances. The importance of the patient's physical state and its implications will be highlighted in subsequent chapters.

## Summary

At 10 weeks following surgery:

(1) A proportion (13.7%) of the sample had difficulties in obtaining their supply of equipment on discharge from hospital.

(2) Three brands of appliance were used by 88% of the sample.

(3) Proportionately twice as many permanent colostomates in non stoma nurse districts were wearing a drainable bag ($P < 0.05$).

(4) Almost one quarter of patients had changed to a different appliance since discharge from hospital, and one quarter of the sample had modified either the way in which they wore their appliance, or the appliance itself.

(5) Problems due to collapse or over-inflation of the bag were of major concern to some patients.

(6) Some patients in the sample had experienced detachment of the bag with spillage (7.6%). Proportionately more of these patients came from non stoma nurse districts ($P < 0.05$).

(7) Self-care in management of appliances was significantly greater in stoma nurse districts ($P < 0.05$).

(8) Scores on the appliance problems scale (APS) were significantly related to age, extent of physical symptoms and type of stoma, but were unrelated to having access to a stoma care nurse.

(9) Scores on the satisfaction with appliance scale (SAS) were significantly and negatively related to physical symptoms and significantly and positively related to having access to a stoma care nurse.

# 8

# Life After Surgery

'I'm not complaining, don't get me wrong,
I'm just glad to be here—singing this song.'

We have already seen that although most patients were not fully recovered from surgery, the majority were managing their own appliances. We have also seen that a few had experienced disasters along the way. In this chapter, we will assess the extent to which patients were beginning to adapt to life with a stoma at 10 weeks following surgery. In doing this, patient responses to three measures will be analysed. The first of these was devised to measure the patient's subjective appraisal of the quality of life compared with his life before surgery. The second was devised to assess the level of his social activities compared with the level before surgery. The third measure is one of psychological adjustment. All these measures are described more fully in Chapter 2.

Abrams (1984) maintains that:

'The goal of successful ostomy surgery is to return the patient to the life-style he enjoyed before his operation and, for those who were living with a chronic illness like ulcerative colitis, to restore them to complete health.' (p. 73)

In Chapter 2 we identified the following factors, which may facilitate or hinder adaptation.

(1) *Age*  Adaptation may be more difficult for older people.

(2) *Physical state*  Patients who are relatively free from symptoms or complications will adapt more readily that those who are not.

(3) *Access to a stoma care nurse*  Patients who have access to a stoma care nurse may adapt more readily that those who do not.

(4) *Permanence of stoma*  Patients who understand that their stoma is temporary may adapt less well than those who have been told that it is permanent.

(5) *Trade off*  Those who have ulcerative colitis or Crohn's disease may consider a stoma as a reasonable trade off for a chronic illness and adapt more

readily. Patients who understand that they have cancer may adapt more readily in the short-term.

(6) *Length of illness*   Patients for whom the onset of illness was sudden may adapt less readily than those who have been ill for some time.

(7) *Marital status*   Patients who have the support of a spouse may adapt more readily than those who do not.

(8) *Sex*   Women may adapt less readily than men.

(9) *Type of admission*   Patients who have emergency surgery may adapt less well than those who undergo elective surgery.

These are the factors that will be examined more closely in analysis.

## Quality of life

The quality of life scale (QLS) assesses the patient's activity level, enjoyment of life and happiness, relative to that experienced before surgery. It is essentially a subjective measure in that the patient makes the appraisal by comparing his present activity level and feelings with those pertaining to his life before he had his operation. A high score on this scale indicates a higher quality of life. A score of 150 would indicate little change in the quality of life compared with before surgery.

The mean (average) score on the QLS across the whole sample was 144.6

**Table 8.1**   Analysis of covariance: quality of life

| Source of variance | Sum of squares | d.f. | Mean square | F |
|---|---|---|---|---|
| *Covariates* | | | | |
| Physical state (SQRT) | 37 199.4 | 1 | 37 199.4 | 12.99*** |
| Age | 65 701.5 | 1 | 65 701.5 | 22.95*** |
| *Main effects* | | | | |
| Access to a stoma nurse | 3 350.3 | 1 | 3 350.3 | 1.17 |
| Temporary/permanent stoma | 15 622.1 | 1 | 15 622.1 | 5.46* |
| Trade off | 20 556.8 | 2 | 10 278.4 | 3.59* |
| Length of illness | 42 299.1 | 2 | 21 149.6 | 7.39** |
| Marital status | 11 083.8 | 1 | 11 083.8 | 3.87* |
| Sex | 1 880.6 | 1 | 1 880.6 | 0.66 |
| Type of admission | 5 026.5 | 1 | 5 026.5 | 1.76 |
| *Error* | 715 685.5 | 250 | 2 862.7 | |

*** $P < 0.001$
 ** $P < 0.01$
  * $P < 0.05$

(s.d. = 59.3). One case is missing from this analysis. The results of covariance analysis of QLS scores are given in Table 8.1. In this analysis QLS scores were adjusted for age and physical state before the remaining factors (2 to 7 above) were fed into the analysis. Each of these factors was then, in turn, adjusted for all other factors.

It can be seen that both age and physical state are strongly related to QLS scores. It must be remembered that as each patient made his subjective appraisal relative to his quality of life before surgery, the relationship with age implies that there is a differential decrease in quality of life for older people following stoma surgery. Moreover, this decrease is still there when differences due to physical state have been partialled out. Similarly, after controlling for age, QLS scores are negatively related to scores on the physical symptoms scale (PSS); the more frequent and severe the patient's symptoms, the lower is his quality of life.

After controlling for age and the extent and severity of physical symptoms the remaining effects can be examined, each of which is controlled for the others. The figures given in Table 8.1 indicate that the most significant effect is that of length of illness. The adjusted QLS scores by length of illness are given in Table 8.1a. Thus, we can see that patients who had been ill for a longer

**Table 8.1a**

|  | QLS adjusted mean score | n | s.d. |
|---|---|---|---|
| Onset less than 1 month's duration | 135.9 | 182 |  |
| Onset between 2 and 3 months' duration | 157.5 | 35 |  |
| Onset greater than 3 months' duration | 169.9 | 45 |  |
| *All* | 144.6 | 262 | 59.3 |

period of time appear to feel that the quality of their lives has improved since surgery.

The next most significant effect relates to whether patients understood that their stoma was temporary or permanent. The adjusted scores for these groups are given in Table 8.1b. Apparently, those patients who understood

**Table 8.1b**

|  | QLS adjusted mean score | n |
|---|---|---|
| Permanent stoma | 152.3 | 148 |
| Temporary stoma | 134.6 | 114 |

that their stoma was temporary were less happy, enjoyed life less and were less active than their counterparts who knew that their stoma was permanent.

It would appear that the notion of 'trade off' is also supported with regard to those patients who have ulcerative colitis or Crohn's disease, but is not supported for those patients who understand that their diagnosis is that of cancer (Table 8.1c). The support of a spouse would also seem to be important (Table 8.1d).

**Table 8.1c**

|  | QLS adjusted mean score | n |
|---|---|---|
| Cancer patients | 134.1 | 54 |
| Ulcerative colitis/Crohn's disease | 174.8 | 19 |
| Other | 144.6 | 189 |

**Table 8.1d**

|  | QLS adjusted mean score | n |
|---|---|---|
| Single/widowed patients | 134.5 | 82 |
| Married patients | 149.2 | 180 |

The remaining effects are not significantly related to QLS scores. After controlling for all other effects QLS scores are only marginally higher for males and for those who have access to a stoma care nurse. None of the two-way interaction effects are significant.

Patients were also asked if there was anything that they used to enjoy doing that they felt that they couldn't do now. Overall, their responses included more than 56 different activities ranging from going to church, singing in a choir, horse riding, flying, wrestling with children, fishing for crabs and butchering sheep! Forty per cent of patients said that there was nothing that they felt they couldn't do, some adding that they hadn't yet tried. However, there was considerable evidence of restriction. Ten per cent of patients said that there were several activities that they felt they could not do. Activities which required physical effort, such as gardening, cycling or housework were mentioned by 19% of patients and physical activities which had a social component, such as swimming, were mentioned by a further 17% of patients. Social activities which required less physical effort, such as going out for a drink, were cited by 6% of patients. A minority of patients mentioned travelling or staying away from home at this early stage. Concern about dress was expressed by several females (5%) and 4% of patients answered that they could no longer enjoy sex.

The notion of 'trade off' for patients who had been suffering from ulcerative colitis or Crohn's disease is illustrated by some of their responses:

'I'm enjoying life for the first time in 10 years.'

'At one time I'd be frightened—I like to talk to people now, I used to go in if I saw someone passing. I feel so well, I feel as I should feel. It's like being reborn.'

There were other patients who had been ill for a short time who saw things from an entirely different perspective:

'Can't go out—it's not the same when you go out among people—you lose some of your confidence. It's a big change, it's not like when you go to a toilet and come out, you see you've got this.'

## Social constraints

The social constraints scale (SCS) assesses the degree to which patients have curtailed or expanded their social activities relative to the number and frequency of their social activities before they had surgery. A high score on this scale indicates a greater degree of social constraint. The same variables as before were entered into a covariance analysis of scores on the SCS. The results of this analysis are given in Table 8.2.

It can be seen that both age and physical state bear strong relationships to SCS scores. After controlling for physical symptoms, older patients had

**Table 8.2**  Analysis of covariance: social constraints

| Source of variance | Sum of squares | d.f. | Mean square | F |
|---|---|---|---|---|
| *Covariates* | | | | |
| Physical state (SQRT) | 10.44 | 1 | 10.44 | 12.31*** |
| Age | 11.15 | 1 | 11.15 | 13.15*** |
| *Main effects* | | | | |
| Access to a stoma nurse | 0.67 | 1 | 0.67 | 0.79 |
| Temporary/permanent stoma | 3.67 | 1 | 3.67 | 4.32* |
| Trade off | 1.45 | 2 | 0.72 | 0.84 |
| Length of illness | 2.04 | 2 | 1.02 | 1.20 |
| Marital status | 0.25 | 1 | 0.25 | 0.29 |
| Sex | 0.34 | 1 | 0.34 | 0.40 |
| Type of admission | 0.09 | 1 | 0.09 | 0.11 |
| *Error* | 211.96 | 250 | 0.85 | |

*** $P < 0.001$
 ** $P < 0.01$
  * $P < 0.05$

reduced their social activities to a greater extent than younger patients and after controlling for age those who had fewer symptoms showed a lower level of social constraints than those who had more symptoms.

After controlling for age and extent and severity of physical symptoms only one effect is significantly related to social constraints. Those patients who understood that their stoma might be temporary had curtailed their social life to a greater extent than those who knew that their stoma was permanent (Table 8.2a). None of the two-way interaction effects was significant.

**Table 8.2a**

|  | Social constraints adjusted mean score | n | s.d. |
|---|---|---|---|
| Patients with a permanent stoma | 10.9 | 148 | |
| Patients with a 'temporary' stoma | 11.17 | 114 | |
| *All* | 11.02 | 263 | 0.96 |

**Psychological adjustment**

The present state examination (PSE) was used to assess the prevalence of anxiety or depression. In these first interviews 25.1% of the total sample were assessed as suffering from anxiety, depression or both. Severe depression was manifest in 6.5% of patients. In stoma nurse districts 22.2% of patients were anxious or depressed, 6.2% were severely depressed. In non stoma nurse districts 31.7% of patients were anxious or depressed, with 9.7% suffering from severe depression. The prevalence of depression at 10 weeks following surgery differed very little between patients with different types of stoma.

Analysis of covariance of scores on the PSE was carried out to clarify the relationship between psychological adjustment and those factors which may hinder or facilitate adaptation. It will be recalled that in Chapter 4 we discussed the possibility that questions relating to satisfaction with information may be tapping some dimension of personality. This additional variable was therefore included in the analysis. The results are given in Table 8.3.

Once again, the most important finding emerging from this analysis is the extremely strong relationship between PSE scores and the extent and severity of physical symptoms. Indeed, when physical state is taken into account, age is unrelated to psychological adjustment.

Having controlled for age, physical symptoms and all other main effects, the next most significant factor associated with psychological adjustment is patient satisfaction with information. Sex and marital status also show a

**Table 8.3** Analysis of covariance: psychological adjustment (PSE)

| Source of variance | Sum of squares | d.f. | Mean square | F |
|---|---|---|---|---|
| *Covariates* | | | | |
| Physical state (SQRT) | 47.963 | 1 | 47.963 | 63.545*** |
| Age | 0.046 | 1 | 0.046 | 0.061 |
| *Main effects* | | | | |
| Access to a stoma nurse | 1.595 | 1 | 1.595 | 2.114 |
| Temporary/permanent stoma | 0.106 | 1 | 0.106 | 0.140 |
| Trade off | 0.011 | 2 | 0.005 | 0.007 |
| Length of illness | 1.174 | 2 | 0.587 | 0.461 |
| Marital status | 3.558 | 1 | 3.558 | 4.714* |
| Sex | 4.217 | 1 | 4.217 | 5.586* |
| Type of admission | 1.648 | 1 | 1.648 | 2.184 |
| Satisfaction with information | 8.011 | 1 | 8.011 | 10.614** |
| *Two-way interactions* | 38.021 | 43 | 0.884 | 1.171 |
| Marital status by sex | 5.960 | 1 | 5.960 | 7.897** |
| Sex by satisfaction with information | 2.814 | 1 | 2.814 | 3.728 |
| *Error* | 156.239 | 207 | 0.755 | |

*** $P < 0.001$
** $P < 0.01$
* $P < 0.05$
[1] A square root transformation was carried out on the PSE scores which were also standardised

significant relationship but access to a stoma care nurse, having a temporary or permanent stoma, the notion of 'trade off', length of illness or type of admission are not significantly related. There is one highly significant interaction effect between marital status and sex. An interaction effect between sex and satisfaction with information just fails to reach the 0.05 level of significance. Further analyses were carried out to clarify these findings and to establish which physical symptoms discriminated between those who were anxious or depressed and those who were not. Symptoms which discriminated between the two groups are shown in Table 8.4.

It can be seen that a far greater proportion of patients who were anxious or depressed were still suffering from pain and/or fatigue at the time of these first interviews. Gastrointestinal upsets were also more common in this group of patients, together with urinary tract infections and backache. Sweating discriminated strongly for men, but not at all for women. Significantly more patients who were anxious or depressed reported slight bleeding of the stoma and that the stoma was noisy. It seems possible that these symptoms, which were often of concern to patients but which are unimportant in terms of the patients' physical condition, may be a manifestation of their anxiety or depression rather than a contributing factor. Similarly, there is no way of

**Table 8.4** Affective disorder: prevalence in relation to physical symptoms

| Symptom present | Anxious or depressed (n = 66) % | Not anxious or depressed (n = 197) % |
|---|---|---|
| Fatigue | 93.9 | 67.5*** |
| Pain | 59.1 | 33.5*** |
| Indigestion | 30.3 | 14.2** |
| Nausea | 18.2 | 5.6** |
| Vomiting | 9.1 | 3.0* |
| Diarrhoea | 31.8 | 18.3* |
| Urinary tract infection | 10.6 | 3.0* |
| Slight bleeding of stoma | 59.1 | 42.1* |
| Noisy stoma[1] | 86.9 | 67.6** |
| Backache | 47.0 | 30.5* |
| *Males only* | n = 28 | n = 115 |
| Sweating | 39.3 (11) | 12.2*** |

$\chi^2$ 1 d.f.
*** $P < 0.001$
** $P < 0.01$
* $P < 0.05$
[1] Bowel stomas only ($n = 243$)

knowing at this early stage to what extent fatigue might be a symptom of depression or a contributing factor. A sensation of rectal fullness did not discriminate between the two groups. It was reported by 67% of those patients who had permanent bowel stomas and who were anxious or depressed, and by 64% of their non anxious or depressed counterparts. Incontinence of urine was reported by 15.2% of anxious or depressed females (bowel stomas only) compared with 5% of those who were not anxious or depressed, but this difference was not statistically significant.

The covariance analysis also showed a significant relationship between sex and marital status and psychological adjustment. This appeared to indicate that females were more anxious or depressed than males and, surprisingly perhaps, that married ostomates were more anxious or depressed that those who were single or widowed. However, in interpreting this finding account must be taken of the highly significant interaction effect between sex and marital status. Further analysis was undertaken to clarify this relationship. The mean z scores calculated for the PSE for males and females according to marital status are illustrated in Figure 8.1.

Figure 8.1 indicates that, whereas single or widowed males have lower scores on anxiety and/or depression than those who were married, the pattern differs for females with widows having slightly lower mean scores and single women having the highest scores. These differences are not nearly so marked as they are for men.

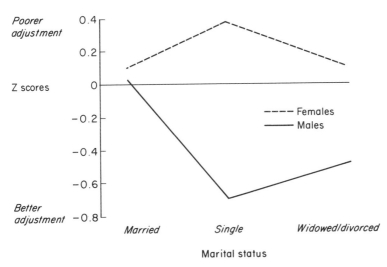

**Figure 8.1**  Psychological adjustment (PSE): z scores by sex and marital status

One other highly significant main effect shown in Table 8.3 is the relationship to satisfaction with information. Those patients who said that there was something else that they would have liked to have been told had higher PSE scores. An interaction effect between sex and satisfaction with information just fails to reach the 0.05 level of significance, but this is worthy of further scrutiny. The results of this analysis are illustrated in Figure 8.2.

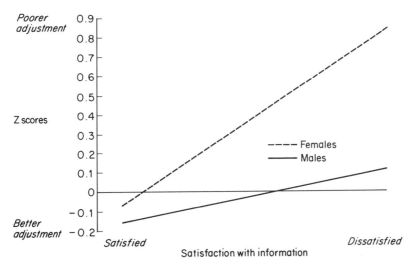

**Figure 8.2**  Psychological adjustment (PSE): z scores by sex and satisfaction with information

It is apparent that, whereas males who would have liked to have been better informed have slightly higher scores on symptoms of anxiety or depression than those who were happy with the information they were given, the difference is most marked for females. Women who were dissatisfied with the information they were given show markedly higher levels of anxiety and/or depression.

The other variables listed in Table 8.3 do not bear a close relationship with psychological adjustment. Although patients in stoma nurse districts have lower scores on average than patients in other districts the difference is not statistically significant when the effects of age, physical symptoms and other factors are partialled out. Whether the stoma is permanent or temporary, whether the patient understands that he has cancer or ulcerative colitis or Crohn's disease, whether he has been ill for a short time or for much longer does not appear to be related to his level of psychological adjustment at 10 weeks after surgery. Patients who had been admitted for emergency surgery did have higher mean scores; 41.7% (10 patients) who had emergency surgery in non stoma nurse districts were assessed as anxious or depressed compared with 26.8% (11 patients) in stoma nurse districts. However, this effect is not statistically significant. Over the sample as a whole, 22.7% of patients who had elective surgery were anxious or depressed compared with 32.3% of those who had emergency surgery.

### The patients' viewpoint

Many patients who were not depressed at the time of these first interviews spoke of being depressed at some point. A few said that they had felt depressed before having their operation, others had felt depressed after surgery or since returning home. Sometimes patients appeared to feel guilty for having such feelings:

> 'It was a nightmare—it's no wonder they kicked me out because I was so depressed.'

> 'I ought to feel ashamed of myself.'

> 'I felt ungrateful to feel miserable.'

A few patients felt that they could have been given more help to overcome their depression:

> 'If they cared on that side a little bit more, probably I would have come out of it you know.'

> 'The attention is not like it used to be—not the staff about, is there?'

> 'I felt as though nobody wanted you—they got the impression I was doing better than I was and then I had a relapse and nobody came.'

Others felt that it might have helped if they had been warned that they might feel depressed:

'That sort of thing wasn't explained.'

Although a few patients were critical others praised staff and were grateful for the patience and understanding they received. For example,

'I just stood there, all trussed up and I couldn't get into the bath. I burst into tears, I felt that helpless and useless. The ward sister was marvellous. She's a woman that's run the ward a long time.'

As one patient so aptly commented:

'It's lots of things that make you depressed.'

Nevertheless, there were several recurring themes in these interviews. One such theme related to inactivity and social limitation:

'I've always been pretty active, I'm losing contact.'

'It's stopped me getting on with what I want to do and as a result I've got a bit depressed.'

'This is no life is it? Just sitting—can't do nothing.'

For some patients pain, illness or exhaustion underlay their depression:

'I feel terrible, depressed and ill, I don't think I would have gone through with it if I'd known. I'm sure I wouldn't.'

'Some days I'm flat down, no sleep, tired and no energy.'

'I've felt so poorly that I tend to feel depressed.'

Some patients expressed feelings of being useless:

'You're only a nuisance, it's no good disguising the fact. I mean—they can't leave me, I'm a prisoner and everybody is held up.'

For some patients the fear of accidents was paramount:

'I've suffered a lot since I had the op. I get tired easily and I just haven't got the confidence in the bag.'

'The two leaks got me a bit depressed.'

Other depressed patients expressed feelings of shame:

'My biggest worry is that it's visible, the wind blowing it up.'

'I feel abnormal and if I thought I was going to have it all the rest of my life it would be very depressing.'

'You feel you are not a woman any more because of the bag.'

Some 'temporary' ostomates were worried about going back into hospital for reversal of the stoma:

'Get on your side again—dreading it. I wondered what the hell he was doing, if only he'd told me.'

'If I could just wake up and have it done without any of those things that you have to go through before you have an op . . . '

Patients also expressed fears about the future:

'I don't feel as though I am making the headway that—I keep having little shooting bits, I get thinking, what the hell is that, you know.'

'They say it was an abscess and they've taken it away but there's some days when I don't feel right and that worries me.'

'I very often think perhaps I shouldn't go to sleep because maybe I'm not going to wake up in the morning and then this black cloud comes over me.'

Five per cent of the sample (11 females and 3 males) said that they had had suicidal thoughts. For example:

'I used to lie awake thinking about the best thing to commit suicide with. Just at times I still get depressed—bags—it doesn't seem natural.'

In contrast to the above, the notion of 'trade off' is illustrated by one ileostomate who said:

'I feel as though I've got my freedom back, I used to get real depressed and down, now it's changed.'

It is important that the above statements are seen in context. Twenty five per cent of the sample were anxious or depressed following surgery from which many were not yet fully recovered. How do these figures compare with those from other studies? In seeking clarification we can look at the prevalence of affective disorder in the general population. We can also look at estimates of the percentage of patients who become depressed following other disfiguring surgery. Finally, we can look at the figures produced by previous studies of ostomates.

Kay et al (1964) conducted a survey of people aged 65 years and over who were identified from the electoral register on Tyneside. They report that 26% of those living at home were suffering from affective disorder. The prevalence was higher for women (29%) than for men (21%). A study of hearing impairment in a sample of 365 old people living at home (Herbst and Humphrey, 1980) revealed a strong relationship between deafness and depression but also showed a strong relationship between age and depression with 31% of people aged 70 to 79 years and 46% of those aged 80 years or more being depressed. These figures were not broken down by sex.

A follow-up study of 75 mastectomy patients, one year after surgery (Maguire et al, 1976) revealed that 17% of women who had undergone this disfiguring operation were suffering from moderate anxiety and/or depression and that a further 8% were suffering from severe anxiety and/or depression. The combined total of 25% is compared with a total of 10% of patients in a control group consisting of women with benign breast disease. The age of the sample is not given.

Kretschmer (1978) suggests that the incidence of persistent, therapy resistant depression for patients with intestinal stomas may be as high as 25%. This is also the figure reported by Devlin et al (1971) following a survey of 120 patients who had had surgery for rectal cancer. A later study of 420 such patients, identified from the South Thames Cancer Registry, was carried out by MacDonald et al (1982). These patients had had surgery between 1958 and 1978 and almost two-thirds of the sample had a permanent colostomy. MacDonald and her colleagues report that 20% of these patients were suffering from limited depression with a further 5% more severely depressed. They also report that patients with a colostomy were no more likely to be depressed than those without, although severe depression was more common among the ostomates. This study also revealed a strong relationship between physical symptoms such as lack of energy, poor sleep, poor appetite and general emotional health. A strong relationship between pain and general emotional health was found only for ostomates. Sex differences were also found in this study; 31% of females were rated as being depressed, compared with 19% of males. The most depressed group comprised women under the age of 65 years of whom 39% were depressed. The least depressed group comprised men over the age of 65 years of whom 18% were depressed.

These studies suggest that approximately one quarter of older people, living at home, suffer from anxiety and/or depression which may also be manifested by one quarter of female patients following disfiguring surgery. It would also seem that women may be more affected than men and that older people may be more prone to affective disorder than younger people, although MacDonald's finding of high levels of depression in younger females runs counter to this suggestion.

Devlin et al (1971) suggest that more work is needed to establish the incidence of depression and its specificity to colostomy in view of the relationship between depression and general disability. The studies of Herbst and Humphrey (1980) and MacDonald et al (1982) give credence to this suggestion which receives further support from the findings reported in this study. Clearly, when differences in psychological adjustment related to physical symptoms are partialled out, there is no significant relationship between age and psychological adjustment. It may, therefore, be that the prevalence of anxiety/depression is directly related to the prevalence of disability which is much greater in older people. This has important implications for studies based on theories of ageing which need to take account of disability levels.

The results of this study and of those described above suggest that women may be more prone to affective disorder than men but these findings also need to be interpreted with caution. For example, it has been suggested that, whereas it is acceptable for women to express their emotions, it is less acceptable for men to do so. It may be that 'denial' is more common among men than among women. This suggestion also receives some support from this study for there is some evidence that men tended to rate themselves as more 'fit' than women. Taking the upper third of the distribution on the physical symptoms scale 23.4% of males described themselves as unwell or seriously incapacitated. In contrast, 36.6% of women in the upper third of the distribution described themselves in this way.

The highly significant finding of greater affective disorder, especially among females who were dissatisfied with the information they had been given, would seem to support the notion that questions relating to satisfaction with information may be tapping the personality dimension of neuroticism. It must be remembered that differences due to physical state and all other factors had been partialled out of the equation. However, the possibility that satisfaction may be related to other factors cannot be ruled out at this stage and will be explored in later analyses.

The finding that married men appear to be more prone to affective disorder than single men or widowers is very difficult to interpret. One possible explanation is that married men find it easier to express their feelings than those who are unmarried. Another possibility is that married men have an additional concern, their relationship with their wife. The PSE contains one question which asks whether there has been any change in this relationship. In response to this question 63.5% of married men said that there had been no change, 6.3% reported a reduction in libido and 30.2% reported a complete loss of libido. These figures can be compared with those for females of whom 68.8% reported no change in their sexual relationship with their husband. It seems doubtful that these differences on one of the 17 items included in the PSE could account for the discrepancy in psychological adjustment between males who were married and those who were not.

Ward sisters and stoma care nurses were asked on interview about their policy with regard to discussion of sexual matters with patients. It became clear that in several of the non stoma nurse districts such matters were never discussed unless they were raised by the patients themselves. In stoma nurse districts, sexual matters were more likely to be discussed although the more commonly adopted approach was to provide an opening for such discussion, usually by asking patients how they thought their husband or wife would feel about them having a stoma. One stoma care nurse said that she asked patients whether they had an active sex life before surgery and commented:

> 'I don't think that as many people have sexual problems as the literature would have you believe.'

Nevertheless, the interviews with patients did reveal that some patients who had not received any counselling on sexual matters might have benefitted from this. For example there were women who no longer felt attractive and there were others of both sexes who felt that sex might be damaging:

'It repels me and I think it's going to repel him.'

'I never used to wear a nightdress but I do now because of the bag, because of the scars, because of the fatness of my tummy. I don't feel attractive at all. I don't feel in the mood.'

'I think he is frightened of hurting me. I could imagine that it would make a mess of it.'

'I am just as keen but I don't want to go and do nothing daft like.'

'I thought afterwards is it—you know—sort of safe at the moment, is it all healed up inside properly.'

Some patients said that they had been too embarrassed to ask about sex possibly because they were older:

'I was too embarrassed to ask. Well probably—maybe because I think at my age someone might turn round and say "Well, good Lord, you must have had your ration", you know.'

'It has been the main problem—I mean it sounds silly at 70 but my dad lived to be 90 and he were courting at 85.'

On the other hand some patients had discussed or asked about their sex lives:

'It's something I was prepared for—it's not the motivation it's the capability that's the problem. The consultant and I agree it is only a question of time.'

Unfortunately, patient questions were not always dealt with sympathetically:

'I asked the nurse and she asked the young doctor and then he went and mentioned it to Mr X and Mr X mentioned it to Mr Y and of course, you know, when you are in bed—surgeon comes, all the students, staff nurse and sister. He says "Oh—she is worried about her sex life." Well I didn't know where to put myself because they all started laughing, you know, I wished I hadn't have asked.'

One male patient with a 'temporary' stoma had postponed his sex life until after he had the stoma reversed. Other patients were gradually adjusting or patiently waiting or hoping that things would return to normal:

'We are conscious about it—the worst thing obviously is that when you decide to make love—I've got to get out of bed, go there, put this thing on and by this time you see we've collapsed laughing. Someone said put a cummerbund type of thing on but—it can't be as spontaneous as it was.'

'My wife laughs about it—we regard it as a bit of a joke. If we had been told it was permanent we wouldn't be so happy about it. At the moment it doesn't bother us.'

## Discussion

The advantages of using covariance analysis to tease out the relationships between the outcome measures and the factors outlined at the beginning of this chapter are clearly apparent. For example it would appear that, whereas age is related to patients' subjective appraisal of the quality of their lives and social constraints, it is unrelated to psychological adjustment when the extent and severity of physical symptoms is taken into account. Indeed, the assessment of patients' physical state has emerged as the single most important variable in each of the analyses.

Although the trend is in the predicted direction, having access to a stoma care nurse is not significantly related to scores on any of the outcome measures after the variance related to other factors is partialled out.

There is evidence of a greater reduction in patients' perceived quality of life for those patients who understand that their stoma is temporary than for those who know that it is permanent. These 'temporary' ostomates also show a greater reduction in their level of social activities. Moreover, we know that these findings obtain after controlling for all other factors including length of illness and type of admission.

The notion of 'trade off' also receives some support, but only with regard to perceived change in quality of life. Patients who know that they have cancer appraise their lives in less positive terms. In contrast, the quality of life is considerably enhanced for those who have ulcerative colitis or Crohn's disease.

The length of time that patients had been ill before surgery is also related to scores on the quality of life measure, but is unrelated to social constraints or to scores on the present state examination.

Marital status is also related to patients' perceptions of their quality of life compared with that experienced before surgery, married patients viewing their lives more positively than those who were single or widowed. However, there is also the finding of a strong tendency for married men to be more psychologically disturbed than those who are unmarried and there is no immediately obvious explanation for this.

The advantages of using analysis of covariance are also illustrated with regard to sex differences. Whereas men had marginally higher scores on perceived quality of life than females, this was not statistically significant and, having controlled for all other variables, there is no evidence to suggest that women reduce their social activities more than men following stoma surgery. This does not of course mean that they engage in as many social activities as men; the measure compares what they do after surgery with what they did before surgery. There is strong evidence to suggest that women have higher levels of affective disorder following stoma surgery than men. This measure is not comparative; it is not known how well adjusted patients were before surgery and it may be that women would have had higher scores at the start. The possibility that findings of sex differences in psychological adjustment may be due, in part, to a greater element of denial by men has already been discussed. The finding that dissatisfaction with information may be linked to psychological adjustment, especially for females, indicates a need for further research to clarify the relationship.

Whereas it was shown in Chapter 4 that the type of admission was related to satisfaction with information given, this variable is unrelated to scores on the outcome measures when all other variables are taken into account.

These findings have considerable implications for nursing practice. We have seen from the interviews with stoma care nurses that they endeavour to tailor their patient care to individual patients and that they correctly identify the elderly and those who are living alone as a group which may require extra care. However, we have seen that the relationship between age and the outcome measures is less strong than that of the patients' physical state. We cannot directly infer that these relationships are causal but the evidence is very strong that the patients' physical state has a bearing on how they perceive their lives, whether they go out or stay in and whether they feel anxious or depressed. A thorough physical assessment is indicated to identify those patients who may be at risk. Those who have more symptoms or more severe symptoms may well be older, but not necessarily so.

It also would seem worth-while to pay more attention to those patients who have temporary stomas to ensure that they do not suspend their life-style while waiting for reversal. For, as will be shown in the next section, the temporary stoma may become permanent and, as one of the surgeons so aptly commented in interview:

'A stoma is for life.'

## Summary

At 10 weeks after surgery the following factors were related to patients' subjective assessment of the quality of life, level of social constraint or psychological adjustment.

(1) *Age* Older patients assessed the quality of their lives significantly less positively than younger patients and also showed greater levels of social constraint.

(2) *Physical state* Patients who had a greater number or more severe physical symptoms assessed the quality of their lives significantly less positively and had significantly higher levels of social constraint than those with fewer or less severe physical symptoms.

(3) *Access to a stoma care nurse* Although the trend was in the predicted direction, having access to a stoma care nurse was not significantly related to quality of life, social constraint or psychological adjustment.

(4) *Permanence of stoma* Patients who understood that their stoma was temporary assessed the quality of their lives significantly less positively and had reduced their social activities to a greater degree than those who

understood that their stoma was permanent. This factor was unrelated to psychological adjustment.

(5) *Trade off*   Patients with ulcerative colitis or Crohn's disease assessed the quality of their lives significantly more positively than other patients. Cancer patients assessed their lives less positively than others. This factor was not significantly related to social constraint or to psychological adjustment.

(6) *Length of illness before surgery*   Patients who had felt really ill for a longer period of time before surgery viewed their lives significantly more positively than those who had been ill for a relatively shorter period. This factor was unrelated to social constraint or to psychological adjustment.

(7) *Marital status*   Patients who had the support of a spouse assessed their lives significantly more positively than other patients. This factor was unrelated to social constraint.

(8) *Sex*   There was no significant difference between males and females with regard to self assessed quality of life or social constraint.

(9) *Sex × marital status*   Married males were significantly more anxious or depressed than unmarried males whereas married females tended to be less anxious or depressed than those who did not have the support of a spouse.

(10) *Satisfaction with information*   Both males and females, but particularly females, who expressed dissatisfaction with the information that they had been given had more symptoms of anxiety and/or depression than those who said that there was nothing else that they would have liked to have been told.

(11) Based on interviews with ward sisters and stoma care nurses it would appear that patients who had sexual problems were less likely to have the opportunity to discuss these in non stoma nurse districts.

# 9

# One Year Later

'I used to lie at night and curse
Hoping that it wouldn't get worse
Then I'd think, "At least I'm here
Even though I've lost some gear".'

## The sample

### Mortality

One hundred and twenty patients were reinterviewed after a period of 1 year. Despite the initial exclusion from the study of patients who had a very poor prognosis, 42 patients died during this time. There was little difference in mortality between patients in stoma nurse districts (14.8%) and patients in non stoma nurse districts (18.4%). Of those who died, 22 had a permanent colostomy, 12 had a 'temporary' colostomy, 3 had an ileostomy and 5 patients had a urinary stoma. The official diagnosis of 6 of those who died is not known. Of the remainder, 35 had a diagnosis of cancer and one patient had ulcerative colitis. The average age of those who died was 65.5 years of age, the youngest was aged 31 years and the oldest was aged 82 years; 20 were male and 22 were female.

### The survivors

The average age of those who were reinterviewed is given separately by type of stoma for patients in stoma nurse districts and non stoma nurse districts in Table 9.1. It can be seen that there are discrepancies in the average age of patients with 'temporary' colostomies, ileostomies and urinary stomas between the two sets of districts. The average age of patients in stoma nurse districts was 63 years, compared with 59.5 years for patients in other districts. The distribution of the sample by sex and marital status is shown in Table 9.2. The distribution of the sexes is very similar for the two sets of districts; 56.4% of patients in stoma nurse districts and 57.1% of patients in the other districts

**Table 9.1** The sample 1 year later. Age: means and standard deviations, by type of stoma and type of district

|  | Stoma nurse districts | | | Non stoma nurse districts | | | All | | |
|---|---|---|---|---|---|---|---|---|---|
|  | n | m | s.d. | n | m | s.d. | n | m | s.d. |
| Permanent colostomy | 41 | 65.9 | 9.8 | 24 | 64.2 | 10.0 | 65 | 65.2 | 9.9 |
| Temporary colostomy | 14 | 71.3 | 10.8 | 6 | 53.3 | 16.4 | 20 | 65.9 | 14.9 |
| Ileostomy | 11 | 43.5 | 18.0 | 9 | 52.4 | 13.7 | 20 | 47.5 | 16.5 |
| Urostomy | 12 | 61.3 | 15.4 | 3 | 55.7 | 18.2 | 15 | 60.2 | 15.5 |
| *Total* | 78 | 63.0 | 14.7 | 42 | 59.5 | 13.1 | 120 | 60.8 | 14.3 |

were male. On the other hand, a larger proportion of patients in non stoma nurse districts was widowed or divorced. The use of analysis of covariance when looking at patient outcome will enable control for the discrepancies in age and marital status between the two sets of districts.

## Stoma reversal

Of the original sample of 105 patients who had a 'temporary' colostomy, 93 survived and 68 of these (73.1%) had their stoma reversed. After a period of one year, 20 patients whose stomas were initially deemed to be 'temporary' were reinterviewed. These patients were asked whether the possibility of reversal had been discussed and how they now felt about this. Their responses are given in Table 9.3.

**Table 9.2** The sample 1 year later: sex and marital status, by type of district

| Type of district | Marital status | Sex | | All |
|---|---|---|---|---|
|  |  | Male % | Female % | % |
| *With stoma care nurses* | | (n = 44) | (n = 34) | (n = 78) |
|  | Single | 9.1 (4) | 11.8 (4) | 10.3 |
|  | Married | 86.4 (38) | 50.0 (17) | 70.5 |
|  | Widowed/divorced | 4.5 (2) | 38.2 (13) | 19.2 |
|  | *Total* | 100.0 | 100.0 | 100.0 |
| *No stoma care nurses* | | (n = 24) | (n = 18) | (n = 42) |
|  | Single | 12.5 (3) | 11.1 (2) | 11.9 |
|  | Married | 70.8 (17) | 50.0 (9) | 61.9 |
|  | Widowed/divorced | 16.7 (4) | 38.9 (7) | 26.2 |
| *Total* |  | 100.0 | 100.0 | 100.0 |

**Table 9.3**  'Temporary' colostomates: attitudes towards reversal 1 year after surgery

| | Stoma nurse districts | Non stoma nurse districts | All |
|---|---|---|---|
| | n | n | n |
| Decision pending: patient still keen | 4 | 1 | 5 |
| Decision pending: patient not keen | 1 | 3 | 4 |
| Stoma now permanent: surgeon's decision | 0 | 1 | 1 |
| Stoma now permanent: patient's decision | 6 | 0 | 6 |
| Stoma reversed and redone | 0 | 1 | 1 |
| Reversal attempted but not done | 3 | 0 | 3 |
| *Total* | 14 | 6 | 20 |

Of the 9 patients who were still waiting for their stomas to be closed, only 5 were still keen to have this done. For example:

'I accept it but I realise there's problems to come. The problem is as I get older it's going to be a mighty problem of changing. I'm losing the use of that finger and I can't grip anything with that. Now I can foresee problems. I'm not senile or anything like that but that is always liable to crop up, isn't it.'

'I mean it was supposed to have been up to 12 weeks. It's dragged out longer, much longer than I thought and I'm still not sure that they are going to reverse it—which is what was in my brain when I said, "Yes I would have it done". But if they tell me don't worry, no matter how long it takes you can have it reversed, I would feel on top of the world and I'd put up with it.'

A further 6 patients, all of whom were in stoma nurse districts, had decided that they would keep their stoma rather than undergo further surgery. For example:

'You've got to go through all that operation again and I wouldn't like that. It's a case of—got used to it.'

'Not at my time of life I can't. The specialist said that it would mean probably 3 weeks in hospital for this to be closed up and then he said at least a month's recuperation. I thought "I don't want to be recuperating a month here on my own, thank you!". So I'm going to keep it.'

Three patients had actually been admitted for reversal although this was not always guaranteed. For example:

'Well, all they could do was resite the colostomy from my right side to my left side and that has made a tremendous improvement. Well, except for having to empty the bag and change it, my life's normal.'

Thus, for the 20 'temporary' colostomates remaining, reversal was still a possibility for only 9 patients of whom only 5 were keen for this to be done.

Three ileostomates in the original sample had also had their stomas reversed. One other ileostomate had had his stoma reversed but following two episodes of obstruction his stoma was recreated.

## Physical symptoms

It will be recalled that at 10 weeks after surgery patients in the larger sample were experiencing a variety of physical symptoms (Chapter 6). Also, it will be recalled that those who were suffering from symptoms such as pain or fatigue were also more likely to be depressed or anxious (Chapter 8). The percentage of patients who were experiencing various symptoms one year postoperatively is shown in Table 9.4. The percentages for these same patients at 10 weeks after surgery are given alongside for comparison.

If the figures for 10 weeks are compared with those for 1 year it will be seen

**Table 9.4** Physical symptoms experienced by patients at 10 weeks and 1 year after surgery

| | Symptoms/complications to some extent | | Symptoms/complications often or severe | |
|---|---|---|---|---|
| | *10 Weeks* | *1 Year* | *10 Weeks* | *1 Year* |
| | (n = 120) | | (n = 120) | |
| | % | % | % | % |
| Fatigue | 70.0 | 46.7 | 13.3 | 8.3 |
| Pain | 38.3 | 35.8 | 8.3 | 10.0 |
| Backache | 29.2 | 35.0 | 5.8 | 11.7 |
| Sweating | 19.2 | 10.8 | 3.8 | 1.7 |
| Indigestion | 17.5 | 24.2 | 2.5 | 4.2 |
| Nausea | 8.3 | 16.7 | 0.0 | 6.7 |
| Vomiting | 10.0 | 13.3 | 2.5 | 2.5 |
| Constipation | 19.2 | 25.8 | 5.0 | 4.2 |
| Diarrhoea | 19.2 | 25.8 | 5.0 | 4.2 |
| Incontinence (urine)[1] | 7.6 | 13.3 | 1.0 | 3.8 |
| Urinary infection | 5.0 | 6.7 | 0.8 | 4.2 |
| Problems–abdominal wound | 3.3 | 1.7 | 1.7 | 1.7 |
| Problems–perineal wound[2] | 29.4 | 15.8 | 2.5 | 5.8 |
| Discharge (other) | 18.3 | 20.8 | 3.8 | 8.3 |
| Prolapse of stoma | 2.5 | 8.3 | 0.0 | 1.7 |
| Retraction of stoma | 9.2 | 5.8 | 1.7 | 3.3 |
| Stenosis of stoma | 1.7 | 0.8 | 0.0 | 0.0 |
| Hernia of stoma | 0.8 | 5.3 | 0.0 | 3.3 |
| Obstruction of stoma | 0.8 | 1.7 | 0.0 | 0.8 |
| Slight bleeding of stoma | 44.2 | 34.2 | 0.0 | 0.8 |
| Severe bleeding of stoma | 0.8 | 0·8 | 0.0 | 0.0 |
| Ulcers of stoma | 3.3 | 3.3 | 0.0 | 0.0 |
| Infection of stoma | 1.7 | 1.7 | 0.0 | 0.8 |
| Flatus[1] | 91.4 | 68.6 | 21.9 | 21.0 |
| Odour | 45.8 | 35.0 | 7.5 | 4.2 |
| Noise[1] | 74.3 | 64.8 | 3.8 | 9.5 |
| Sensation of rectal fullness[2] | 55.3 | 61.2 | 9.4 | 11.8 |

[1] Bowel stomas only (n = 105)
[2] Permanent bowel stomas only (n = 85)

that, although fewer patients were suffering from fatigue, almost one half of the sample still complained of tiredness one year after surgery. The percentage of patients who said that they had pain or backache was almost the same, amounting to approximately one third of the sample.

Problems with the abdominal wound were infrequent but 15.8% of those who had abdominoperineal excision of the rectum said that their perineum was still painful or discharging.

Other less serious symptoms, though reduced in frequency, were still experienced by many patients. For example, approximately two-thirds of the sample complained of flatus or noise and more than one third of the sample said that smell was a problem to some extent. A sensation of rectal fullness was still experienced by 61% of the sample.

Some symptoms were more prevalent than before. The percentage of patients experiencing gastrointestinal symptoms was greater than at 10 weeks following surgery. Similarly, the percentage of patients who said that their stoma had prolapsed (8.3%) or that they had a hernia near the stoma was also greater (5.8%). Of the 20 patients whose stoma was originally deemed to be 'temporary', 3 said that it had prolapsed, 2 said that it had retracted and 1 said he had a hernia. Of the 65 surviving permanent colostomates, 5 complained of prolapse, 3 of retraction, 2 were experiencing episodes of obstruction and 5 said that they had a hernia. Of the 20 ileostomates 1 said that the stoma prolapsed, 2 complained of retraction and 1 of stenosis. One patient with a urinary stoma said that he had a hernia.

Problems such as these can cause severe distress to patients as illustrated by one woman with a retracted ileostomy who was waiting to see the surgeon with a view to readmission:

> 'My stoma retracts and I get a lot of burst leaking bags. I went to town with my son and we had a bit of lunch and I said to him "I'm going to the loo for a minute" and when I got there I had a burst, so we had to walk three-quarters of a mile to the car park and I was walking along padded up with toilet paper. Now when that sort of thing happens your self confidence goes out of the window.'

### Readmissions

Other patients had already been readmitted to hospital since the first interviews, sometimes more than once. The percentages are given in Table 9.5. The figures given in Table 9.5 show that 40% of patients had been readmitted to hospital on at least one occasion and that 11.6% of patients had been admitted more than once. It can also be seen that the percentage of patients who had been readmitted to hospital is slightly higher in stoma nurse districts although the average number of readmissions per patient is lower (0.55) than in non stoma nurse districts (0.67). Thirty-nine per cent of colostomates, 40% of ileostomates and 47% of patients with a urinary stoma had been readmitted. The reasons for each readmission are given separately by type of

**Table 9.5**　Percentage (and numbers) of readmissions, by type of district

| Number of readmissions per patient | Stoma nurse districts (n = 78) % | Non stoma nurse districts (n = 42) % | All (n = 120) % |
|---|---|---|---|
| 0 | 57.7 (45) | 64.3 (27) | 60.0 |
| 1 | 32.0 (25) | 21.4 (9) | 28.3 |
| 2 | 7.7 (6) | 7.1 (3) | 7.5 |
| 3 | 2.6 (2) | 4.8 (2) | 3.3 |
| 7 | 0.0 | 2.4 (1) | 0.8 |
| *Total* | 100.0 | 100.0 | 99.9 |

**Table 9.6**　Reasons for readmission by type of district

| | Stoma nurse districts (n = 33) | Non stoma nurse districts (n = 15) | All patients (n = 48) |
|---|---|---|---|
| Reversal | 1 | 1 | 2 |
| Obstruction | 2 | 2 | 4 |
| Stoma surgery for a second time | 1 | 1 | 2 |
| Reversal (not done) | 2 | 0 | 2 |
| Excision of rectum | 2 | 1 | 3 |
| Refashioning/resiting of stoma | 3 | 1 | 4 |
| Chemotherapy/radiotherapy | 0 | 7 | 7 |
| Pain therapy | 6 | 1 | 7 |
| Tests | 1 | 1 | 2 |
| Abscess/fistula/sinus | 7 | 4 | 11 |
| Metabolic instability | 2 | 0 | 2 |
| Ascites | 1 | 1 | 2 |
| Excision of tumour | 1 | 1 | 2 |
| Bladder/kidney problems | 3 | 4 | 7 |
| Penile implant | 1 | 0 | 1 |
| Prostatectomy | 3 | 0 | 3 |
| Hernia | 1 | 0 | 1 |
| Orthopaedic surgery | 2 | 0 | 2 |
| Cardiovascular problems | 4 | 2 | 6 |
| Stretching of anus | 0 | 1 | 1 |
| Admissions (*n*) | 43 | 28 | 71 |

district in Table 9.6. When looking at the figures given in Table 9.6, it is important to remember that some patients had more than one admission. For example, two patients had their stoma reversed but were later readmitted for obstruction and had stoma surgery for a second time. One patient was admitted for chemotherapy at monthly intervals for a period of 6 months. One colostomate who had been admitted twice for 'bladder warts' was waiting to go into hospital for a third time for further treatment. Rather more patients were admitted for treatment of an abscess, fistula or perineal sinus than for any other reason. Refashioning or resiting of the stoma had been performed on four colostomates, and the woman who had retraction of her ileostomy was waiting for admission. Two urostomates had been admitted for 'metabolic instability'. Seven patients had been admitted for problems such as haematuria, retention and catheterisation or kidney failure following radiotherapy.

Ten of the admissions in stoma nurse districts and two of the admissions in the other districts appear to be unrelated to the previous stoma surgery. For example, two patients were admitted for orthopaedic surgery, one of whom had a hip replacement. Three patients had a prostatectomy and another had an operation for a 'double hernia'. Six patients had been readmitted for cardiovascular problems such as a 'heart attack', thrombosis, or aneurism.

One urostomate had a penile implant and was not very happy with the result. He complained that after standing for half an hour his testicles became 'rock hard' but he also had problems when sitting:

> 'I definitely wish I hadn't had it. Well, when I walk a lot it's always—when I'm sat down with ordinary women, they think I'm getting frisky so that's why I'm always conscious of it and I'm like this, my hands are always—like this because there is a distinct showing there you know.'

## Issues that patients wanted to discuss

In these second interviews patients were asked whether there had been times during the past year when they would have liked to be able to discuss things with someone. They were then asked what they would have liked to discuss and whether they had done this. Almost two-thirds of the sample said that there were things that they had wanted to discuss; their responses are categorised in Table 9.7. By far the largest category relates to physical problems. Thirty-five per cent of patients were concerned about such things as incontinence, urinary infection, anal discharge, rashes, diarrhoea, the effects of chemotherapy or radiotherapy, backache, pain, itching, herniation, constipation, chest pain and a variety of other problems.

The second largest category relates to stoma management and equipment. More than 1 in 10 patients would have liked to discuss stoma care problems such as retraction or protrusion of the stoma, leakage or skin irritation. Others had wanted more information on the equipment available.

Five patients had wanted to discuss psychological problems. For example, one patient whose husband had just died could not accept her stoma. Another patient was distressed when someone he knew had stoma surgery and died 3 months later. The patient was concerned that he had been unable to help.

Another five patients said that they had wanted to discuss sexual problems and the same number said that they had wanted to discuss how other

**Table 9.7** Topics that patients would have liked to have discussed over a 12 month period

| Discussed: | Stoma nurse districts | | Non stoma nurse districts | | All districts | | Total sample (n = 120) | |
|---|---|---|---|---|---|---|---|---|
| | Yes | No | Yes | No | Yes | No | | |
| | n | n | n | n | n | n | n | % |
| Health/physical problems | 24 | 3 | 13 | 2 | 37 | 5 | 42 | 35.0 |
| General issues/ information | 0 | 0 | 2 | 0 | 2 | 0 | 2 | 1.7 |
| Stoma care/ equipment | 6 | 5 | 2 | 2 | 8 | 7 | 15 | 12.5 |
| Psychological problems | 2 | 0 | 2 | 1 | 4 | 1 | 5 | 4.2 |
| Sex | 4 | 0 | 1 | 0 | 5 | 0 | 5 | 4.2 |
| Work | 1 | 0 | 0 | 0 | 1 | 0 | 1 | 0.8 |
| Other ostomates | 3 | 0 | 0 | 2 | 3 | 2 | 5 | 4.2 |
| *Total* | 40 | 8 | 20 | 7 | 60 | 15 | 75 | 62.6 |

ostomates felt and wanted to know how they could help others who were going through the same experience.

Were these needs catered for? The figures given in Table 9.7 suggest that, for the most part, patients had discussed these issues. When patients were asked with whom they had talked they named a variety of personnel. Their responses to this question are summarised separately for the two sets of districts in Table 9.8.

The proportion of patients who consulted their GP is very similar between the two sets of districts. Almost one third of all patients who had things that they wished to discuss had done so with their GP. General practitioners were

**Table 9.8** Percentage personnel with whom patients discussed their problems

| | Stoma nurse districts (n = 48) | | Non stoma nurse districts (n = 27) | | All (n = 75) | |
|---|---|---|---|---|---|---|
| | n | % | n | % | n | % |
| Stoma care nurse | 19 | 39.6 | 0 | 0.0 | 19 | 25.3 |
| Stoma care nurse from elsewhere | 0 | 0.0 | 2 | 7.4 | 2 | 7.4 |
| Company nurse | 0 | 0.0 | 4 | 14.8 | 4 | 5.3 |
| Surgeons | 7 | 14.6 | 4 | 14.8 | 11 | 14.6 |
| General practitioner | 15 | 31.2 | 8 | 29.6 | 23 | 30.7 |
| Established ostomate | 1 | 2.1 | 0 | 0.0 | 1 | 1.3 |
| Relatives/friends | 5 | 10.4 | 2 | 7.4 | 7 | 9.3 |
| Not discussed problem | 8 | 16.7 | 7 | 25.9 | 15 | 20.0 |
| *Total* | | 114.6* | | 99.9 | | 109.2* |

* Some patients discussed their problems with more than one person

**Table 9.9** Personnel contacted by patients for help with stoma in 6 months before the second interview

| | Stoma nurse districts (n = 78) | | Non stoma nurse districts (n = 42) | | All (n = 120) | |
|---|---|---|---|---|---|---|
| | n | % | n | % | n | % |
| Stoma care nurse | 26 | 33.3 | 0 | 0.0 | 26 | 21.7 |
| Ward nursing staff | 0 | 0.0 | 4 | 9.5 | 4 | 3.3 |
| District nurse | 1 | 1.3 | 0 | 0.0 | 1 | 0.8 |
| Company nurse | 2 | 2.6 | 2 | 4.8 | 4 | 3.3 |
| Surgeons | 6 | 7.7 | 3 | 7.1 | 9 | 7.5 |
| General practitioner | 3 | 3.8 | 3 | 7.1 | 6 | 9.0 |
| No one | 47 | 60.3 | 33 | 78.6 | 80 | 66.7 |
| *Total* | | 109.0 | | 107.1 | | 112.3* |

* 15 patients contacted more than one person

more frequently approached with regard to physical problems, but patients in stoma nurse districts often discussed these with stoma care nurses also. In fact the major difference between the two sets of districts lies in the proportion of patients who discussed their problems with the stoma care nurse. Clearly, she was the major sounding board for patients who had access to her services. On the other hand some patients in non stoma nurse districts discussed their problems with a company nurse or with a stoma care nurse from elsewhere.

Patients were asked whether they had contacted anyone for help with their stoma in the 6 months prior to the second interview. The figures given in Table 9.9 are based on the full sample. Taken as a whole, one third of all patients had contacted at least one person for help with their stoma in the 6 months before they were interviewed. However, the proportion of those who did so was considerably greater in stoma nurse districts. In other districts, some patients contacted ward sisters or other nursing staff. A minority of patients in both sets of districts had sought help from company nurses. Interpretation of the discrepancy between the two sets of districts in the proportion of patients who sought help is somewhat difficult. It may be that if a stoma care nurse is not available patients tend to persevere in isolation rather than bother their GP. For example:

'Well, when it first started to protrude I thought well I won't go bothering the doctor because the stoma nurse had said like "Any problems, give me a ring".'

It is also possible that fewer patients in non stoma nurse districts needed help or realised that they might be helped.

In these second interviews patients were again asked whom they considered had been of most help to them since their discharge from hospital. Their responses to this question are summarised in Table 9.10.

**Table 9.10**   Personnel considered to have been most help to patients since discharge from hospital

|  | Stoma nurse districts (n = 78) % | Non stoma nurse districts (n = 42) % | All (n = 120) % |
|---|---|---|---|
| Spouse | 28.2 | 45.2 (19) | 34.2 |
| Other relative | 19.2 | 9.5 (4) | 15.8 |
| Friends/neighbours | 5.1 | 2.4 (1) | 4.2 |
| Stoma care nurse | 28.2 | 0.0 | 18.3 |
| Company nurse | 1.3 | 9.5 (4) | 4.2 |
| District nurse | 2.6 | 9.5 (4) | 5.0 |
| General practitioner | 12.8 | 14.3 (6) | 13.3 |
| Surgeon | 2.6 | 4.8 (2) | 3.3 |
| Established ostomate | 2.6 | 0.0 | 1.7 |
| Other | 2.6 | 0.0 | 1.7 |
| Patient himself | 3.8 | 4.8 (2) | 4.2 |
| No one particularly | 5.1 | 9.5 (4) | 6.7 |
| Total | 114.1* | 109.5* | 112.6* |

\* Some patients cited more than one person

When this question was put to patients in the first interviews, proportionately fewer patients named their GP and proportionately more patients named their spouse (Table 6.1). In these second interviews, the major difference between the two sets of districts lies in the percentage of patients who said that their husband or wife had been of most help. Moreover the figures are somewhat misleading as a greater proportion of patients in non stoma nurse districts were widowed. Whereas 39.3% of married patients in stoma nurse districts named their spouse, 73.1% of married patients in non stoma nurse districts did so. In these districts a greater proportion of patients also said that the district nurse, or a company nurse, had been of most help to them since their discharge from hospital.

Only two patients, both in stoma nurse districts, said that another established ostomate had been of most help, yet it will be recalled that in the first interviews 17% of patients who had not been visited by someone who had had stoma surgery in the past said that they would like a visit. We also saw that many ward sisters and stoma care nurses said that they would arrange such visits if patients so wished. To what extent, therefore, had these patients, who had lived with a stoma for more than a year, been approached with a request to visit other patients? Twenty-four patients (17.5%) said that they had been asked if they would be willing to visit other patients but only 14 had actually done so. Seven colostomates and 3 patients with urinary stomas had visited other patients in hospital and 3 colostomates and 1 urostomate had visited other patients in their own homes. However, these visits were not always initiated by professionals:

'My daughter rang me one day and said could this lady ring me. She had just come out of hospital and she was feeling terribly depressed. So I said "Well yes, of course, if I can help I will". She rang me up and she was on the phone about an hour and she said at the end of the time she felt much better. Then she said "If ever you come into . . . would you please come and see me". So my daughter fetched me on purpose and I was with her about 2 hours.'

Other people were contacted and asked to visit by hospital staff:

'They rang me and asked me to go and see a lady, she was very low and she wouldn't eat. There was a mark on her bed, well, you know, they stitch up your backside and she said, "I haven't made that mess" and I said, "You have, love, because I made them myself." And she said, "Who are you?" I told her I'd had a colostomy. She said "You've got a colostomy!" and I said, "Yes and I swim, I dance and I drink whisky!" She started to laugh and she said, "You haven't had a colostomy" and I said "Yes, love, and I've got a bag on my side". Well she started to take an interest and she said "Oh, I thought everything was going wrong". I said "No, everything is going right". Now, I took a bag, because the bag they give in hospital is a drainage one and I took her a small delicate one which I don't care for but it's delicate for a woman and I said, "You can even use those." It lifted her—"Oh," she said, "I feel lovely". I went to see her the next day and she was eating and she was happy.'

One ostomate was asked to visit a patient at home before he was due to go into hospital for surgery:

'He seemed to be rather apprehensive about it. I was with him for about an hour and gave all the pros and cons and I thought I got him—fairly satisfied. Subsequently there was a phone call from his daughter to ask if I'd go and have another talk with him because he'd had the operation and apparently he was very depressed.'

If contact with other ostomates is beneficial one would expect that patients would get in touch with one of the self-help groups such as the Ileostomy Association. In the first interviews, one quarter of the sample expressed an interest in contacting one of these organisations, however only 12.5% of those who were reinterviewed had done so. A further 25% said that they were interested.

## Discussion

In the first interviews we saw how those patients who had 'temporary' stomas viewed their lives less positively and had curtailed their social lives to a greater extent than those who had to accept that their stoma was permanent. We now see that one quarter of surviving 'temporary' ostomates still had their stoma 1 year later. The implications of this for nursing care are only too apparent; it is clearly important that at least as much effort needs to be made to encourage the 'temporary' ostomate to accept life with a stoma as is made to encourage those whose stomas are known to be permanent.

At 10 weeks following surgery we also saw that the patient's physical state was the most important variable relating to his perceived quality of life, psychological adjustment and social activity. The extent to which patients were still suffering from various physical symptoms is therefore a rather depressing feature of these second interviews. Similarly, a large number of patients had been readmitted to hospital, sometimes more than once, in the period which had elapsed since the first interviews.

It would seem that the majority of patients who had problems that they wished to discuss had been able to discuss them with someone, but it is also interesting to note that more than half of these patients wanted to discuss physical problems and that they were rather more likely to approach the stoma care nurse, if one was available, than their GP. In tandem with this we find that, whereas the proportion of patients who considered that their GP had been of most help to them over the past year is very similar between the two sets of districts, a far greater proportion of married patients in non stoma nurse districts considered that their spouse had been of most help. In stoma nurse districts the stoma care nurse and the spouse ranked equal first. It would seem that, when the help of a stoma care nurse is not available, patients rely more heavily on informal support.

Despite the different impression gained when interviewing care staff, the data obtained in this study suggest that the practice of asking established ostomates to visit patients is very limited. Previous research (Mitchell, 1980) indicated that more than 4 out of 5 colostomy patients who were visited in hospital felt better as a result, and Trainor (1982) found that established ostomates who visited new patients showed significantly greater acceptance of their own stoma. It would seem that there is a potential source of help for new patients that is relatively untapped. There are, of course, drawbacks to the use of such visitors. The first is the advisability of using visitors, when either the visitor or the new patient has a poor prognosis, for the survivor may be subjected to further distress. The second drawback is that unless the visitor is exceptionally well informed about the appliances that are available the patient may not be given good advice. The greatest benefit that an established ostomate has to offer is that of enabling a new patient to realise that it is possible for patients to have a life which is 'normal' in most respects.

In this chapter it has been shown that one third of the sample had sought help with stoma care during the 6 months before these second interviews. In the next chapter we will take a second look at patients' problems and satisfaction with their appliances.

## Summary

(1) One hundred and twenty patients were reinterviewed of whom 85 had colostomies, 20 had ileostomies and 15 had urinary stomas.

(2) Forty-two patients had died since the first interviews and 72 patients had had their stoma reversed. Nine patients were still waiting for stoma reversal but only 5 were keen to have this done.

(3) More than 1 year following surgery, 27% of patients who originally understood that their stoma was temporary still had their stoma.

(4) The most frequently reported symptoms were fatigue, pain, backache, flatus, noise, smell and, for those with permanent bowel stomas, a sensation of rectal fullness.

(5) Forty per cent of patients had been readmitted since the first interviews, 11.6% more than once.

(6) Of the 37 patients who had been employed 2 months before having stoma surgery, 21 were working 1 year after surgery, 7 were still off work, 1 was unemployed and 6 had retired. The mean time off work was 24 weeks for ileostomates and patients with urinary stomas and 18 weeks for colostomates.

(7) Almost two-thirds of the sample had things that they wished to discuss during the year following surgery. Physical problems predominated.

(8) Forty per cent of the patients in stoma nurse districts had sought help with their stoma in the six months before being reinterviewed. Twenty-one per cent of patients in other districts had done so.

(9) In stoma nurse districts the stoma care nurse and a spouse were considered to have been of most help since patients were discharged from hospital. In other districts a greater proportion of patients said that their spouse had been of most help.

# 10

# One Year Later: Stoma Management

'"He" has an independent way,
I can't control him through the day
But if he wasn't here with me
I might not be here, too, you see.'

### Stoma care equipment

At 10 weeks after surgery, some patients appeared to be using appliances that might not be considered entirely appropriate. On reinterview, it was found that 19.2% of patients in stoma nurse districts and 28.6% of patients in non stoma nurse districts had changed to a different appliance. Nevertheless, only 14.2% had actually changed the make of appliance that they used; the same three brands dominated the market and were used by 85% of ostomates. Most patients gave several reasons for changing to a different appliance. Eight patients changed for reasons of skin sensitivity or leakage. In stoma nurse districts more than half of those who changed did so on the recommendation of the stoma care nurse. In non stoma nurse districts one half of those who changed did so on the recommendation of a company nurse or a stoma care nurse from elsewhere.

In these second interviews, details were obtained of all the stoma care products that were being used by these now established ostomates. These are listed separately in Table 10.1 by type of stoma.

Clearly, the majority of colostomates appeared to favour a closed bag. However, it is interesting to note that proportionately fewer colostomates in stoma nurse districts were using a drainable appliance (16%) than in non stoma nurse districts (33%). Two of the 20 ileostomates remaining in the sample, both of them in non stoma nurse districts, were using closed bags.

Almost three-quarters of urostomates appeared to prefer a 2-piece appliance compared with just over a quarter of patients with bowel stomas. Rather more patients with urinary stomas also wore belts and used extra tape. One urostomate had invented his own night drainage system:

**Table 10.1**　Stoma care products being used by patients 1 year following surgery

|  | Colostomy (n = 85) % | Ileostomy (n = 20) % | Urostomy (n = 15) % |
|---|---|---|---|
| 1-piece drainable bag | 18.8 | 65.0 (13) | 26.7 (4) |
| 1-piece closed bag | 45.9 | 5.0 (1) | 0.0 |
| 2-piece drainable bag | 3.5 | 25.0 (5) | 73.3 (11) |
| 2-piece closed bag | 24.7 | 5.0 (1) | 0.0 |
| Drainable and closed bags | 2.4 | 0.0 | 0.0 |
| Irrigation equipment | 4.7 | 0.0 | 0.0 |
| Stoma cap | 7.1 | 0.0 | 0.0 |
| Night drainage system | 0.0 | 0.0 | 93.3 (14) |
| Belt | 9.4 | 10.0 (2) | 40.0 (6) |
| Filter | 65.9 | 45.0 (9) | 0.0 |
| Additional wafer | 7.1 | 25.0 (5) | 6.7 (1) |
| Extra tape | 7.1 | 25.0 (5) | 33.3 (5) |
| Bag covers | 9.4 | 15.0 (3) | 13.3 (2) |
| Skin gel/creams | 32.9 | 35.0 (7) | 33.3 (5) |
| Lotions | 3.5 | 10.0 (2) | 0.0 |
| Koraya paste | 16.5 | 15.0 (3) | 6.7 (1) |
| Deodorant drops | 23.5 | 30.0 (6) | 6.7 (1) |
| Deodorant spray | 28.2 | 40.0 (8) | 0.0 |
| Powder | 11.8 | 15.0 (3) | 0.0 |
| Solvent | 1.2 | 5.0 (1) | 0.0 |
| Wipes | 3.5 | 15.0 (3) | 6.7 (1) |
| Cutter | 1.2 | 0.0 | 0.0 |
| Microenema | 1.2 | 0.0 | 0.0 |

'It's just a commercial polythene holder which used to have detergents in. I drilled a hole in the top and put the tube through, pushed it tight. I put it in a bucket at the side of the bed—just to steady it. I have two of them and alternate weeks I change it and clean it out with vinegar and hot water.'

Filters were used by approximately two-thirds of colostomates but by just under one half of ileostomates. Additional wafers, deodorant drops and air fresheners were more commonly used by ileostomates than by colostomates, but skin preparations were used by approximately one third of all patients.

One female and three male colostomates had been taught to irrigate their stomas. Three were between the age of 45 and 55 years but one patient was 75 years old. One man in a non stoma nurse district who had been having problems with leakage and was waiting to be readmitted for 'leakage from the wound' was taught to irrigate by a stoma care nurse from elsewhere:

'She seemed to be quite keen to promote this sort of thing so I gave it a try and it's funny but it gives me a feeling that I've got some control over the situation. It's psychological perhaps. I have the odd accident now and then but I suppose that's only to be expected.'

The other three patients who practised irrigation were in stoma nurse districts.

One had been admitted for refashioning of a retracted stoma but said that this had not been very successful. Another patient was concerned about her stoma which worked continuously:

'I knew my nurse felt for me because I was different to all her other patients, they seemed to go twice a day and that was it. She suggested the idea to me and of course I was thrilled at the thought of it. I wasn't quite so thrilled when I saw the equipment but I was prepared to have a go because—well—I got very depressed about it. I was pleased, the first thing I noticed was my stomach went down. I was aware that once I'd got my colostomy I didn't have a flat tummy, but this seemed to make me—different, I felt different.'

Two other patients also occasionally used a stoma cap. One man liked to wear one for various activities, including swimming, but felt that his needs were not fully understood:

'I know they are being questioned but if the doctors understood it was a psychological—they look at it as if it is a luxury but it's not, it's a necessity for someone like me. It's just that some of the doctors can't just b . . . well take it in. I'm a happy healthy man and when I ask for these, I only ask for 50 a year and they are not a luxury, they're for my mind.'

It will be recalled that at 10 weeks following surgery, 13.7% of patients said that they had had some difficulty in obtaining their supply of equipment. This question was repeated in these second interviews when 13 patients (10.8%) said that they had experienced some problems. Four patients said that there was a long delay before their order was completed. Four patients said that they had been unable to get the correct appliance. Three patients said that there had been some confusion relating to the prescription and two patients had to make two trips to the chemist which was several miles away.


## Stoma management

In these second interviews patients were asked about their bathroom facilities. The majority of patients had a toilet in the bathroom (71.7%). Just over one quarter of patients had a separate toilet (25.5%). Only one patient had to contend with an outside toilet which didn't have any lighting. Although this patient did have a bathroom, it did not have a toilet and was said to be very cold. This particular patient changed his appliance in the kitchen. All patients had access to a bath (69.2%), a shower (5.8%) or both (25%). Bathroom heating was said to be inadequate by 14.2% of the sample overall.

At 1 year following surgery, 95.8% of ostomates were fixing their own appliances, although 10 patients (9.2%) said that they had help in doing this. The main reasons for requiring help with the appliance were disabilities such as poor sight (7 patients) or the position of the stoma (3 patients). Four patients received help for reasons of preference and 1 patient had her appliance changed by residential care staff.

All patients were asked about the amount of time that they spent caring for their stoma and changing appliances. Of the 4 patients who practised irrigation, 3 spent more than 60 minutes in the bathroom each day and one patient spent an average of between 30 and 45 minutes. Of the remaining 116 patients 83.6% spent less than 30 minutes in the bathroom per day, 12.1% spent between one half and three-quarters of an hour and 3.4% spent between three-quarters and 1 hour. Only 1 patient, who had an ileostomy, seemed to spend a great deal of time in stoma management: an average of 106 minutes per day.

The percentage of patients who had modified their appliance in some way and the types of modification made were very similar to those reported for the first interviews and will not be repeated here.

In contrast, the proportion of patients who had experienced some sort of disaster with their appliance was proportionately greater than that reported before. However, it must be remembered that a year had elapsed since the last interviews. Seventeen patients (14.2%) described such an episode which had occurred during the past year.

## Satisfaction with appliance

In the framework for evaluation (Chapter 1) we saw how satisfaction with appliance was one factor which might facilitate adaptation to life with a stoma. Unfortunate episodes such as those outlined in Chapter 7 cannot be expected to promote confidence in a bag. On the other hand, some patients had changed to a different appliance since the first interviews and, presumably, found their new appliance more to their liking.

In the last chapter, there was discussion about how a minority of patients had developed some form of stomal complication such as retraction, prolapse, stenosis, parastomal hernia, infections or episodic obstruction. It seems reasonable to suppose that complications such as these could make stoma management more difficult.

The appliance problems scale (APS) and the appliance satisfaction scale (ASS) were readministered in the course of these second interviews. A correlation of 0.4 was obtained between scores on the APS at 10 weeks after surgery and 1 year later. For the SAS, 10 week scores correlated 0.53 with scores obtained 1 year later. A correlation of $-0.58$ was obtained between scores on the two scales.

Analysis of covariance was used to assess patient outcome based on these two measures. Those patients who practised irrigation were omitted from these analyses. The following variables were fed into the analysis:

(1) age;

(2) physical state;

(3) access to a stoma care nurse;

(4) type of stoma;

(5) experience of severe leakage such as a 'burst' bag;

(6) stomal complications;

(7) change to a different appliance.


The appliance problems scale (APS)

It will be recalled that higher scores on this scale indicate greater problems. The results of covariance analysis are given in Table 10.2.

The patient's physical state is still strongly related to problems with appliance 1 year after surgery as shown in Table 10.2. However, after controlling for physical state, it would appear that age is unrelated to problems with appliance.

It would also appear that scores on this scale are unrelated to having access to a stoma care nurse, to stomal complications or to having changed to a different appliance. On the other hand, APS scores are significantly related to the type of stoma that a patient has. For example the mean (average) score for the 116 patients included in the analysis is 7.05 (s.d. = 1.65). The mean score for the 20 ileostomates is 7.65, the mean score for the 81 colostomates is 6.7 and the mean score for patients with urinary stomas is 7.93. When adjusted for age, physical state and all other factors the difference between these scores is reduced but, as indicated in Table 10.2, it is still highly significant ($P < 0.003$).

**Table 10.2** Analysis of covariance: appliance problems 1 year after surgery

| Source of variance | Sum of squares | d.f. | Mean square | F |
|---|---|---|---|---|
| *Covariates* | | | | |
| Physical state (SQRT) | 31.34 | 1 | 31.34 | 15.21*** |
| Age | 5.37 | 1 | 5.37 | 2.61 |
| *Main effects* | | | | |
| Access to a stoma nurse | 1.32 | 1 | 1.32 | 0.64 |
| Type of stoma | 24.74 | 2 | 12.37 | 6.00** |
| Burst bag | 22.25 | 1 | 22.25 | 10.80** |
| Stomal complications | 2.02 | 1 | 2.02 | 0.98 |
| Change of bag | 5.68 | 1 | 5.68 | 2.76 |
| *Error* | 220.2 | 107 | 2.06 | |

\*\*\* $P < 0.001$.
  \*\* $P < 0.01$.
   \* $P < 0.05$.

One other factor, that of experiencing a 'burst' bag, is also significantly related to scores on the APS ($P < 0.001$). The adjusted mean score for those who had experienced such a disaster is 8.14 compared with an adjusted mean score of 6.84 for their more fortunate counterparts.

None of the two-way interaction effects was significant.

### The satisfaction with appliance scale

It will be recalled that higher scores on this scale indicate greater satisfaction. The results of analysis of covariance are given in Table 10.3. It would appear that the extent and severity of patients' symptoms is also related to their satisfaction with appliances. Having controlled for physical state, age is not significantly related to scores on the SAS. Having controlled for both age and physical state, patients in stoma nurse districts have higher scores on this scale, but the difference is not statistically significant.

When looking at the other main effects, it is important to take the finding of significant interaction effects into account. For example, it would seem that satisfaction with appliance is unrelated to the type of stoma that a patient has when this is considered in isolation. However, it is related to the type of stoma when considered in conjunction with stomal complications. The mean score on this scale for the whole sample is 322 (s.d. = 55); the mean score for those

**Table 10.3** Analysis of covariance: satisfaction with appliance 1 year after surgery

| Source of variance | Sum of squares | d.f. | Mean squares | F |
|---|---|---|---|---|
| *Covariates* | | | | |
| Physical state (SQRT) | 49 397.2 | 1 | 49 397.2 | 24.38*** |
| Age | 2 921.0 | 1 | 2 921.0 | 1.45 |
| *Main effects* | | | | |
| Access to a stoma nurse | 5 701.6 | 1 | 5 701.6 | 2.81 |
| Type of stoma | 2 097.2 | 2 | 1 048.6 | 0.52 |
| Burst bag | 9 411.1 | 1 | 9 411.1 | 4.65* |
| Stomal complications | 14 794.6 | 1 | 14 794.6 | 7.30** |
| Change of bag | 6 742.7 | 1 | 6 742.7 | 3.33 |
| *Two-way interactions* | 68 959.3 | 14 | 4 925.7 | 2.43** |
| Type of stoma × stomal complications | 25 947.2 | 2 | 12 973.6 | 6.40** |
| Burst bag × change of bag | 9 572.3 | 1 | 9 572.3 | 4.72* |
| Stomal complications × change of bag | 17 605.3 | 1 | 17 605.3 | 8.69** |
| *Error* | 188 436.1 | 93 | 2 026.2 | |

*** $P < 0.001$.
** $P < 0.01$.
* $P < 0.05$.

who had stomal complications is lower for each type of stoma but is especially low for the nine ileostomates who had some form of stomal complication (230).

There is a further interaction effect between stomal complications and change of appliance. In the absence of stomal complications there is no difference in satisfaction with appliance between those who changed to a different bag and those who did not. For those with stomal complications there is a considerable difference in satisfaction according to whether they had changed to a different appliance. For those who had changed, the mean score is 323 but for those who had not changed to a different type of appliance the mean score is 282.

The third significant interaction effect is between the experience of a 'burst' bag and change of appliance. The mean scores for those ostomates who had not experienced a disaster with their appliance is almost the same whether or not they had changed to a different type of appliance. For those who had been unfortunate enough to experience a disaster satisfaction with appliance is far lower if they had not changed to a different bag.

### Discussion

It is somewhat disquieting to find that 1 in 10 of these now established ostomates had had difficulty in obtaining equipment and that more than 1 in 10 had experienced some episode of severe leakage. The finding that such episodes were related to scores on the appliance problems scale (APS) suggests that these disasters were associated with other appliance problems. The finding that, unless they had changed to a different bag, those who had experienced disaster were far less satisfied with their appliance, underlines the lack of confidence experienced by patients following such an episode. The presence of stomal complications also makes for a lower level of satisfaction with appliances especially for ileostomates.

On a more optimistic note, it should be noted that scores on the APS were lower than at 10 weeks following surgery, indicating that patients were now having fewer problems with their appliances. Similarly, scores on the SAS were higher, indicating that satisfaction had increased. It seems unlikely that this is due to a test effect as this was not found in the test/retest reliability study (Chapter 2).

There was no difference between the two sets of districts with regard to scores on the appliance problems scale (APS) or the satisfaction with appliance scale (SAS). Thus, the difference in satisfaction with appliances which was evident at 10 weeks following surgery had disappeared 1 year later. However, we have to consider also the finding that a greater proportion of ostomates in non stoma nurse districts had changed to a different appliance and that more than one half had done so on the advice of a company nurse or a stoma care nurse from elsewhere.

In an article written in 1984 Devlin, referring to colostomates, stated that:

> 'All English patients who can irrigate are now taught to do so. Contraindications to irrigation include arthritis, blindness and peristomal hernia.' (p. 1016)

In the light of this statement it is surprising to find, in this study, that so few colostomates practised irrigation (4.7%). Indeed, when asked, many patients said either that it had not been discussed, or that they had not previously heard about irrigation. We have seen how one patient liked to wear a stoma cap whilst swimming. This same patient shredded his used appliances into extremely small pieces before flushing them down the toilet. The reason that he did this was so that he could emerge from the toilet 'just like anyone else'.

The market for stoma care equipment, dominated by three companies, is a very lucrative one worth approximately £40 million per annum. It may not be in the interests of these companies to promote irrigation, but it seems possible that substantial savings to the NHS might be possible if:

- stoma care nurses were made accountable for their budget. (When interviewed later, 9 of the 12 stoma care nurses said that they didn't have a budget allocation, and 2 said that they felt sure that they had but that they didn't know what it was. Only 1 stoma care nurse said that she had been asked to keep a check on her spending.)
- greater attention were to be given to the possibility of irrigation for those patients who are suitable and who might, if they knew about it, actually prefer this method.

According to Devlin (1984), lack of confidence in the appliance and the fear of accidents are major reasons for social isolation and withdrawal. In the next chapter we will examine the social and psychological consequences of stoma surgery.

### Summary

(1) Of the total sample, 22.5% had changed to a different appliance during the previous year.

(2) One half of those who had changed to a different appliance did so on the recommendation of a stoma care nurse or a company nurse.

(3) Irrigation was practised by 4.7% of colostomates.

(4) With regard to appliance management, 95.8% of ostomates were totally independent.

(5) Of all the patients, 14.2% had experienced at least one episode of severe leakage.

(6) Covariance analysis revealed that scores on the appliance problems scale (APS) were significantly related to the extent and severity of physical symptoms, to having experienced an episode of severe leakage and to type of stoma.

(7) Covariance analysis revealed that scores on the satisfaction with appliance scale were significantly related to the extent and severity of physical symptoms. Satisfaction with appliance was lower for those who had stomal complications, especially ileostomates. For those who had complications or who had experienced an episode of severe leakage, satisfaction was higher if they had changed to a different appliance.

(8) There was no significant difference in scores on either the appliance problems scale (APS) or the satisfaction with appliance scale (SAS) between patients in stoma nurse districts and those elsewhere.

(9) Scores on the appliance problems scale (APS) and the appliance satisfaction scale (ASS) indicated that, in general, patients were having fewer problems and were more satisfied with their appliances than at 10 weeks after surgery.

(10) Of the 12 stoma care nurses interviewed only one said that she was accountable for her budget.

# 11

# Patient Adaptation

'I'm stuck with "Esra" for a while,
He's back to front so do not smile,
Although he is a mucky lad,
He's really not so very bad.'

In the last chapter we saw that, although some patients were still having problems with their appliances, the overall level of problems was reduced compared with the problems experienced at 10 weeks after surgery and the overall level of satisfaction with appliances was higher. In this chapter, we will look at how well patients had adapted to life with a stoma. Adaptation is defined in terms of patients' subjective appraisal of the quality of their lives, the degree to which they had resumed their social activities, their psychological adjustment and their attitudes towards the stoma.

### Variables included in covariance analysis

In the first chapter, several factors were identified which might facilitate or hinder adaptation. At 10 weeks after surgery, we examined the relationship between these factors and the scales devised to assess patient outcome. The number of variables that can be included in covariance analysis is limited, especially when the sample size is small. Moreover, after a period of one year some of the original variables are less relevant. For example, most of the 'temporary' stomas had been reversed and, because many of the 'temporary' ostomates had been admitted for emergency surgery, the number of these patients is also much reduced. These two variables are, therefore, omitted from these later analyses.

The notion of 'trade off' which was supported at 10 weeks after surgery but only with regard to patients who had ulcerative colitis or Crohn's disease is also omitted as the number of these patients is rather small (15) and they can be looked at separately.

The following variables are included in covariance analysis:

(1) *Age* Adaptation may be more difficult for older people.

(2) *Physical state*   Patients who are relatively free from symptoms may adapt more readily than those who are not.

(3) *Access to a stoma care nurse*   Patients who have access to a stoma care nurse may adapt more readily than those who do not.

(4) *Sex*   Women may adapt less readily than men.

(5) *Marital status*   Patients who have the support of a spouse may adapt more readily than those who do not.

(6) *Length of illness*   Patients who have been ill for some time may adapt less readily than those for whom the onset of illness was sudden.

## Quality of life

A correlation of 0.56 (Pearson r) was obtained between scores on the QLS at 10 weeks after surgery and 1 year later.

It must be remembered that when patients were asked to complete this scale they were asked to appraise their enjoyment of life, activity level and happiness relative to how they felt *before* surgery. A score of 150 would indicate no change in the quality of life and a higher score would indicate an improvement. The mean score on the QLS for the whole sample is 158.2 (s.d. = 58.6). This compares with a mean of 152.6 (s.d. = 63.8) for these same patients at 10 weeks after surgery. The mean score on the QLS for the 15 patients whose diagnosis was that of ulcerative colitis or Crohn's disease is 207.9 (s.d. = 71.9). This would seem to indicate that, on average, these patients feel that their quality of life had greatly improved since having stoma surgery, but the size of the standard deviation suggests that this is not so for all these patients.

The results of covariance analysis of QLS scores are given in Table 11.1. In this analysis QLS scores were adjusted for age and physical state before the remaining factors were fed into the analysis. Each of these factors was then adjusted for all other factors. Two-way interactions were adjusted for covariates, main effects and other two-way interactions. Three-way interactions were adjusted for covariates, main effects, two-way interactions and other three-way interactions. This model explains 33% of the variance. The figures given in Table 11.1 indicate that both age and physical state are strongly related to patients' subjective appraisal of the quality of their lives. Moreover, the relationship between each of these variables and QLS scores is that which is unique to that variable. In other words, older patients and those with high levels of physical symptoms view their lives less positively than before surgery, whereas those who are younger or have fewer symptoms view their lives more positively. Essentially this is a repeat of the pattern which was found at 10 weeks postoperatively.

**Table 11.1**  Analysis of covariance: quality of life 1 year after surgery

| Source of variance | Sum of squares | d.f. | Mean square | F |
|---|---|---|---|---|
| *Covariates* | | | | |
| Physical state (SQRT) | 40 896.3 | 1 | 40 896.3 | 20.59*** |
| Age | 21 259.0 | 1 | 21 259.0 | 10.70** |
| *Main effects* | | | | |
| Access to a stoma nurse | 1 283.2 | 1 | 1 283.2 | 0.65 |
| Length of illness | 25 004.6 | 1 | 25 004.6 | 12.59*** |
| Marital status | 435.9 | 1 | 435.9 | 0.22 |
| Sex | 3 777.9 | 1 | 3 777.9 | 1.90 |
| *Two-way interactions* | 11 771.3 | 6 | 1 916.9 | 0.96 |
| Sex × marital status | 8 397.2 | 1 | 8 397.2 | 4.23* |
| *Error* | 212 554.4 | 107 | 1 986.5 | |

*** $P < 0.001$.
** $P < 0.01$.
* $P < 0.05$.

After controlling for both age and physical state, only one of the main effects is significant. The mean score on the QLS for those patients who had been ill for more than 3 months before surgery is significantly higher than the mean score of those for whom the onset of illness was more abrupt. After controlling for other variables the mean score of patients in stoma nurse districts is not significantly different from that of patients in the other districts.

One significant two-way interaction effect between sex and marital status is also shown in Table 11.1. The results of further analysis to clarify this relationship are shown in Figure 11.1. It would appear that, whereas there is little difference in the appraisal of the quality of their lives between males and females who were married, there is a very large difference between the sexes for those who did not have the support of a spouse. Both widowed and single men viewed their lives far more positively than married men. In contrast, widowed or single females viewed their lives far less positively than married females and also less positively than before surgery.

Following their response to the visual analogue scale assessing 'happiness', which forms part of the QLS, patients were asked why they were more or less happy than they were before surgery. The responses of patients who scored in excess of 65, or below 35 points, on this scale were subsequently divided into five categories. Forty-three patients scored 65 or more on the scale and of these 16 made statements to the effect that they were happier because their health had improved. For example, they felt better or they were free from pain. Twelve patients made statements which suggested that their morale had improved. Either they were no longer worried about their illness, had been told that they were cured, felt more content or had a greater appreciation of

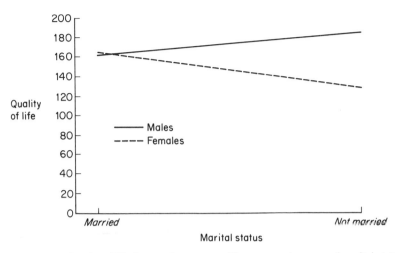

**Figure 11.1**   Quality of life 1 year after surgery. Mean scores by sex and marital status

life. Ten patients made statements suggesting that they were happier because they were free from bowel/bladder problems. Three patients said that their social life had improved and two patients said that they were happier because they had a new or enhanced relationship.

Eighteen patients scored below 35 points on the 'happiness' scale. Seven made statements relating to social restrictions which they attributed to ill health. Interpersonal relationships was the next biggest category accounting for five patients two of whom had been bereaved. Four patients made comments which showed that they had not been able to come to terms with life with a stoma. Two patients said that they were less happy because they were in pain.

### Social constraints

A correlation of 0.48 (Pearson r) was obtained between scores on the social constraints scale (SCS) at 10 weeks after surgery and 1 year later.

It will be recalled that a score on the SCS which is in excess of 10 indicates a reduced level of social activity compared to that enjoyed before surgery. A score of 10 would indicate exactly the same level of activity as that enjoyed before surgery. A score of less than 10 indicates a higher level of social activity than before surgery.

The mean score on the SCS for the whole sample of 120 patients is 9.32 (s.d. = 1.6) indicating a considerable reduction on the mean score of 10.94 (s.d. = 0.93) for these patients at 10 weeks after surgery and an overall rise in the average level of social activity compared with that obtaining before surgery.

**Table 11.2** Analysis of covariance: social constraints 1 year after surgery

| Source of variance | Sum of squares | d.f. | Mean square | F |
|---|---|---|---|---|
| *Covariates* | | | | |
| Physical state (SQRT) | 19.38 | 1 | 19.38 | 9.45** |
| Age | 0.19 | 1 | 0.19 | 0.09 |
| *Main effects* | | | | |
| Access to a stoma nurse | 1.07 | 1 | 1.07 | 0.52 |
| Length of illness | 17.11 | 1 | 17.11 | 8.35** |
| Marital status | 0.01 | 1 | 0.01 | 0.00 |
| Sex | 0.11 | 1 | 0.11 | 0.05 |
| *Two-way interactions* | 47.41 | 6 | 7.90 | 3.85** |
| Sex × marital status | 8.13 | 1 | 8.13 | 3.97* |
| Length of illness × marital status | 22.04 | 1 | 22.04 | 10.75** |
| Access to a stoma nurse × marital status | 10.24 | 1 | 10.24 | 5.00* |
| *Error* | 219.17 | 107 | 2.05 | |

*** $P < 0.001$.
** $P < 0.01$.
* $P < 0.05$.

The results of analysis of covariance of scores on the SCS are given in Table 11.2. This model explains 29.3% of the variance. It can be seen that the extent and severity of patients' symptoms is strongly related to scores on this scale. After controlling for physical state, age does not appear to be related to SCS scores.

Length of illness is the only main effect which is significant, however there is an interaction effect between this variable and marital status. Further analysis was carried out to clarify this relationship. The results are shown in Figure 11.2.

The mean score on the SCS for those patients who had been ill for a longer period of time before surgery is lower than the mean score for patients who were ill for a shorter period indicating a relatively greater increase in social activity. This explains the finding of a significant main effect and is a logical finding as this scale uses patients as their own controls and those who had been ill for a longer period had probably reduced their level of social activity before surgery. Married patients who had been ill for more than 3 months before having surgery had increased their social activities to a far greater extent than their counterparts who were not married (Figure 11.2). The situation is reversed for patients who had been ill for less than 3 months; those who were not married had increased their social activities to a greater extent than their married counterparts.

After controlling for other variables the mean score on this scale for patients in stoma nurse districts is not significantly different from the mean

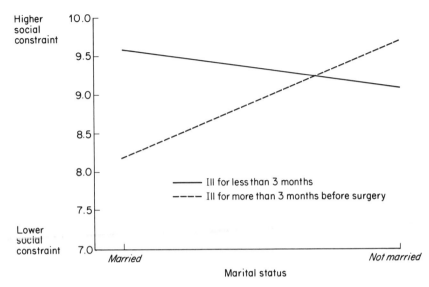

**Figure 11.2** Social constraint 1 year after surgery. Mean scores by marital status and length of illness before surgery

score for patients in other districts. However, there is also an interaction effect between marital status and having access to a stoma care nurse. Further analysis was undertaken to clarify this relationship. The results of this analysis are illustrated in Figure 11.3.

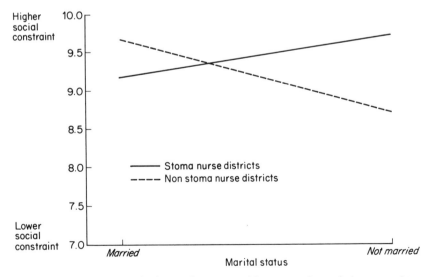

**Figure 11.3** Social constraint 1 year after surgery. Mean scores by marital status and type of district

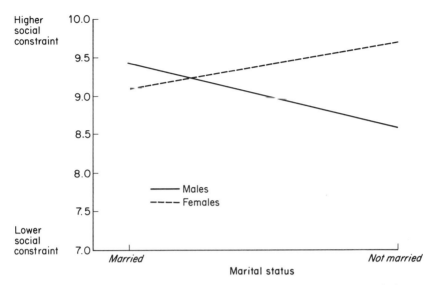

**Figure 11.4**   Social constraint 1 year after surgery. Mean scores by sex and marital status

There was little difference in mean scores between patients in stoma nurse districts and patients in non stoma nurse districts or between those who were married and those who were not. However, Figure 11.3 indicates that, in non stoma nurse districts, patients who were not married had increased their social activities to a greater extent than those who were married. On the other hand, in stoma nurse districts married ostomates had increased their social activities to a greater extent than those who were single or widowed.

Marital status is involved in one other interaction effect. The results of analysis to clarify the relationship between sex and marital status are shown in Figure 11.4. The highest score on social constraints is for women who were single or widowed, whereas the lowest is for men who were single or widowed (Figure 11.4). The difference between males and females who were married is very much smaller.

## Relationship with spouse

It would seem that marital status is quite important but that its relationship with social constraints is quite complex. Towards the end of the interviews patients were asked whether the operation had made any difference to their relationship with their spouse. Of the 81 married ostomates 39.5% said that they felt closer, 54.3% said that their relationship was the same and 6.2% said that they felt further apart. There was very little difference between the two sets of districts; however there was a tendency for rather more men than women to say that they felt closer to their spouse (41.8% compared with 34.6%) and for rather more women than men to say that they felt further apart (11.5% compared with 3.6%). These differences are not statistically significant.


## Holidays

A holiday is often an important social event. Now that more than 1 year had elapsed since surgery, patients were asked whether they usually went away for a holiday. Sixteen patients responded by saying that they never went away for holidays, 11 patients said that they sometimes went on holiday, but not every year, and 93 patients said that they always or nearly always went away for a holiday. Patients were then asked if they had taken a holiday since they had stoma surgery. Their responses to this question are given in Table 11.3.

It is apparent that almost two-thirds of those patients who said that they went away for a holiday every year or most years had been away for a holiday since having stoma surgery. The figure was higher for patients in stoma nurse districts (68.9%) than for patients in other districts (59.4%). Less than 1 in 5 of those patients who usually took a holiday gave stoma surgery as a reason for not taking a holiday during the previous year, but some of these were actually planning to take a holiday. For example:

'I wasn't well enough but I've got confidence now.'

'Not this year but I'm going on three holidays next year.'

'I'm saving up for a holiday, we are looking forward to it.'

One major hurdle for some ostomates was the problem of bag disposal while they were away from home:

'It's not easy unless you have a toilet attached to your bedroom.'

For some patients this hurdle was one that they were not prepared to tackle:

**Table 11.3** Percentage (and number) of ostomates who had taken a holiday away from home since surgery

| | | Holiday since surgery | | | |
|---|---|---|---|---|---|
| Holiday before surgery | n | Yes % | No (surgery) % | No (other reason) % | All % |
| Yes/most years | 93 | 64.5 (60) | 19.4 (18) | 16.1 (15) | 100.0 |
| Sometimes | 11 | 45.5 (5) | 9.1 (1) | 45.5 (5) | 100.0 |
| No | 16 | 6.3 (1) | 0.0 (0) | 95.7 (15) | 100.0 |
| All | 120 | 55.0 (66) | 15.8 (19) | 29.2 (35) | 100.0 |

'I don't want to be bothered changing the bag in somebody else's home.'

Others had worried about it beforehand but had gone away despite this apparent problem. For example:

'I managed OK. I washed them, wrapped them up and put them in a bin in a public convenience.'

Another patient wrote to the Ileostomy Association to ask for their advice.

On a more positive note it did seem that for some ostomates taking a holiday put the seal of acceptance on their stoma. For example:

'I managed perfectly well on holiday—I've decided to keep it.' (i.e. decided against reversal)

'I was very worried about flying before but not now. My hobby is aviation, I've been on a trip to London to go in a helicopter, I've been on Concorde and I've flown 12 times in the past year. I'm going to China in 2 weeks.'

One patient had been to Spain for 3 months and another patient went to Jerusalem with her daughter on the spur of the moment:

'I couldn't have gone if I hadn't had a plentiful supply of bags.'


## Other restrictions

Towards the end of these second interviews patients were asked if there was anything that they used to enjoy doing that they felt that they couldn't do now. Sixty-three ostomates (52.5%) mentioned at least one restriction and four ostomates (3.3%) said that there were several activities which they could no longer enjoy. The most commonly restricted activities were those which entailed physical effort but also had a social component (18.3%). Swimming is one such activity which was specifically mentioned by 5.8% of patients.

The second biggest category included purely physical activities such as gardening, joinery and housework. Activities such as these were mentioned by 13.3% of ostomates.

Purely social activities were mentioned by a further 5% of patients and 5% said that they felt that they could not travel or stay away from home.

Five ostomates (4.2%) said that they could no longer enjoy sex, 2 patients (1.7%) said that they could no longer enjoy passive activities such as knitting and 1 patient (0.8%) said that she could no longer dress as she used to do.


## Psychological adjustment

The present state examination (PSE) was also administered in these second interviews. A correlation of 0.46 was obtained between scores on the PSE obtained in first and second interviews.

Over the whole sample, 23.3% of patients were either anxious or depressed. Anxiety or depression was more common among females (32.7%) than among males (16.2%). Severe depression was present in 5.8% of patients. The figures are very similar for the two sets of districts. In stoma nurse districts, 24.4% of patients were anxious or depressed including 6.4% who were severely depressed. In non stoma nurse districts, 21.4% (9 patients) were anxious or depressed including 4.8% (2 patients) who were severely depressed.

Of the 20 patients whose colostomies were originally deemed to be 'temporary', 8 (40%) were assessed as being anxious or depressed. This may be compared with 21.5% of the 65 patients with permanent colostomies. Of the 20 ileostomates, 4 (20%) were anxious or depressed. Only 2 of the 15 patients with urinary stomas (13.3%) were assessed as anxious or depressed. As will be shown later, 15 of the 28 ostomates who were anxious or depressed were among those who said that they were still unable to accept their stoma.

As in the first interviews, a covariance analysis was conducted to clarify the relationship between scores on the PSE and patient attributes. The results of this analysis, which explain 40% of the variance, are given in Table 11.4. The figures given in Table 11.4 indicate, yet again, the strength of the association between affective disorder and the extent and severity of physical symptoms. Having controlled for physical state, age is unrelated to scores on the PSE.

Length of illness before surgery is the only significant main effect. Those who had been ill for a longer period of time appeared to be less prone to psychological disorder. Of course this group includes many of the patients who had ulcerative colitis or Crohn's disease.

**Table 11.4**  Analysis of covariance: psychological adjustment[1] 1 year after surgery

| Source of variance | Sum of squares | d.f. | Mean square | F |
|---|---|---|---|---|
| *Covariates* | | | | |
| Physical state (SQRT) | 38.49 | 1 | 38.49 | 57.45*** |
| Age | 0.33 | 1 | 0.33 | 0.49 |
| *Main effects* | | | | |
| Access to a stoma nurse | 0.01 | 1 | 0.01 | 0.01 |
| Length of illness | 2.84 | 1 | 2.84 | 4.24* |
| Marital status | 0.45 | 1 | 0.45 | 0.67 |
| Sex | 0.41 | 1 | 0.41 | 0.61 |
| *Two-way interactions* | 4.60 | 6 | 0.77 | 1.15 |
| Sex × marital status | 2.52 | 1 | 2.52 | 3.76 |
| *Error* | 71.87 | 107 | 0.67 | |

*** $P < 0.001$
** $P < 0.01$
* $P < 0.05$
[1] A square root transformation was performed on the PSE scores which were also standardised

There is one interaction effect between sex and marital status which just falls short of the 0.05 level of significance. Further analysis to clarify this indicates that, whereas there is little difference between females who are married and those who are not married, there is a considerable difference between males who are married and those who are single or widowed. Unmarried males appear to be less prone to affective disorder. Essentially, this is a repeat of the pattern obtained at 10 weeks after surgery.

Further analysis was undertaken to find out which physical symptoms were related to affective disorder. Those symptoms which are significantly related to the presence or absence of anxiety and/or depression are given in Table 11.5.

It is useful to compare the list of symptoms appearing in Table 11.5 with the list of symptoms which were related to anxiety and/or depression at 10 weeks following surgery (Table 8.4). Several symptoms appear in both lists. These include fatigue, pain, backache, indigestion, nausea, vomiting and urinary infection. Diarrhoea, slight bleeding of the stoma and sweating (males) which were related to affective disorder at 10 weeks following surgery are not significantly related 1 year later. On the other hand, there are symptoms which are significantly related to psychological adjustment at 1 year following surgery which were unrelated at 10 weeks. These include incontinence of urine, flatus and odour.

The finding that flatus, noise and odour are more frequently reported by those patients with affective disorder is of considerable interest, but it is

**Table 11.5**  Affective disorder: prevalence in relation to physical symptoms 1 year after surgery

|  | Anxious or depressed (n = 28) % | Not anxious or depressed (n = 92) % |
|---|---|---|
| Fatigue | 71.4 (20) | 39.1** |
| Pain | 60.7 (17) | 17.9** |
| Backache | 50.0 (14) | 30.4* |
| Indigestion | 50.0 (14) | 17.4*** |
| Nausea | 32.1 (9) | 11.9* |
| Vomiting | 17.9 (5) | 4.4* |
| Urinary tract infection | 17.9 (5) | 3.3** |
| Incontinence-urine[1] | 26.9 (7) | 8.9* |
| Flatus[1] | 88.5 (23) | 60.8* |
| Noisy stoma[1] | 80.8 (21) | 58.2* |
| Odour | 67.9 (19) | 25.0*** |
| Sensation of rectal fullness[2] | 75.0 (12) | 60.9 n.s. |

*** $P < 0.001$
** $P < 0.01$
* $P < 0.05$
[1] Bowel stomas only (n = 105)
[2] APER only (n = 80)

impossible to say whether patients who are anxious or depressed tend to be more concerned about these stoma-related symptoms, thus reporting them more frequently, or whether these symptoms are actually more frequent and contribute to their anxiety or depression. Either or both of these explanations may be true.

The interview transcripts of those who were assessed as anxious or depressed revealed a variety of concerns. Twelve patients were worried about their health, 2 were having further investigations, 3 were experiencing severe pain and 4 had abscesses or fistulae. For example:

'If anything goes wrong, or I feel ill or get any pains, this is what I think about.' (cancer)

'I don't feel well, it's stopped me going places.'

'I've had so much pain, it's not the surgery or the stoma, my health has gone down.'

Eight patients expressed concern related to their stoma, 2 had a prolapsed stoma, 4 were concerned about management and 2 about odour or noise:

'It always happens when everybody stops talking.'

Other patients were concerned about family problems such as bereavement or marital discord. One patient expressed feelings of severe loneliness and one was worried about getting a job.

Some of these patients had more than one problem. For example, one man had angina, a fistula and a prolapsed stoma. Another had severe arthritis, could not walk and her husband was an alcoholic.

One patient was still hoping for his stoma to be reversed whereas another was quite glad that this was not going to happen:

' I don't feel as depressed as I was before I got to know that I wasn't having it put back.'

Two patients made more positive comments: one who had symptoms of anxiety and tension simply said that he felt 'fine' and another commented:

'My quality of life has improved because I got very near to taking all my pills. I still wish that I hadn't had it but, then again, I'm glad I can do a lot more.'

One patient out of the sample of 120 had had suicidal thoughts during the month before the interview.


Loss of libido

Only 2 of these anxious or depressed patients spontaneously mentioned that they were concerned that their sex lives were 'finished', but 10 of the 11 men included in this group were married and all of these said that they had complete loss of libido. In contrast, only 12 out of 33 married men who were not anxious or depressed said that they had complete loss of libido and a further 3 said that they had some loss. Care needs to be taken in interpreting this finding as the question about libido is included as part of the psychological assessment. However, if this question were omitted from the PSE the number of anxious or depressed males would have been reduced by one. Loss of libido was also reported by 4 out of the 7 married women who were anxious or depressed and by 4 out of 17 married women who were not anxious or depressed.

## Medication

Following the psychological assessment, patients were asked whether they were taking any tablets to help them sleep or for their 'nerves'. Six of the 28 patients who were anxious or depressed said that they were taking 'nerve' tablets, and 9 said that they were taking sleeping tablets. Only 3 of the 92 patients who were not anxious or depressed were taking medication for their 'nerves' and 19 were taking tablets to help them sleep. Unfortunately, more detailed information on patients' medication was not obtained.

## Acceptance of stoma

The person who wrote the poem at the beginning of this chapter appears to have come to terms with his stoma. These second interviews with patients revealed that some had not accommodated quite so well. When asked whether they had accepted their stoma, patients responded with comments such as, 'I've accepted it', 'I've learned to live with it', I've got used to it', to 'Sadly no', or 'I hate it'. Altogether 26.9% of females (14) and 19.1% of males (13) said that they were unable to accept their stoma. Extremely negative reactions were expressed by 8 patients (6.7%). Acceptance was higher for those who were married (81.5%) than for those who were single or widowed (69.2%), however the majority of these were women. Acceptance was also higher among those with permanent colostomies (81.5%) than among those whose colostomies were originally deemed to be 'temporary' (70%). Five of the 20 ileostomates, 4 of whom had diagnoses of ulcerative colitis or Crohn's disease, and 4 of the 15 patients with urinary stomas said that they had been unable to come to terms with having a stoma.

In stoma nurse districts, 74.4% said that they had accepted their stoma, and in other districts 83.3% of patients said that they had accepted their stoma. These differences are not statistically significant.

Almost one third of those who reacted negatively to their stoma when they first saw it after surgery were still unable to accept it after more than one year had elapsed, and we have already seen 15 of the 27 who could not accept their stoma were anxious or depressed.

These patients also took a less rosy view of the quality of their lives compared to other patients. The mean score on the QLS was 122.3 (s.d. = 55.0) compared with 170.1 (s.d. = 46.1) for those who had accepted their stoma, but there were some patients who scored extremely low. For example one man who had described himself as very active before surgery and had a QLS score of 39 said:

> 'They never told me beforehand that I was going to have a stoma. The thing that worries me is the fact that I feel as if I'm a burden to my wife. If I didn't have this nagging pain in my legs and back—if I didn't have that and I could get out and walk about freely—I think probably you know the answer would be OK, 100%.'

There were others who scored very highly on the QLS. For example, one ileostomate with a diagnosis of Crohn's disease acknowledged that her life had greatly improved in many respects, yet she felt unable to accept her stoma:

> 'It sounds very conceited, although I've had four children—when I was young I was called 'the body' and I was always very proud of my body and figure and I feel flawed. But I can live with it. I think if I'd been 30 and had it done it would have been worse but in 2 years' time I shall be 60 so it doesn't matter so much. I still wish I hadn't had it. I'm glad because I can do a lot more than I could do and I can go places I couldn't before. In one way I am extremely pleased and in another way I am very sad about it.'

When asked why she was very much more happy than she was before surgery this same woman replied:

> 'I don't have the cloud hanging over me—that I am going to make a mess in some shop or in the street or bed or in the house and bathroom or anywhere. I have a lot more confidence.'

In a similar way four other patients who had been unable to come to terms with having a stoma also viewed their lives in a much more positive way than before surgery. It seems possible that patients such as these were still going through a period of mourning, as described by Barney (1978), but that they might eventually adapt to life with a stoma.

There is also evidence that some of these patients who could not accept their stoma had greatly increased their social activities. The mean score on the SCS for these 27 patients was 9.4 (s.d. = 1.9) which is only marginally higher than that for the whole sample. However, scores on the SCS ranged from 4.0 (indicating an enormous increase in social activity compared with before surgery) to 12.0 (indicating a large reduction in social activity). Some of these patients had high levels of physical symptoms which, as we have seen, is strongly related to social constraint, quality of life and affective disorder. Thus, it may be that for some patients their stoma may be perceived as a physical manifestation of their decline in health.

Table 11.6 Employment status before surgery, 10 weeks and 1 year after surgery

|  | Before surgery | | After surgery | |
|---|---|---|---|---|
|  | 2 months | 2 weeks | 10 weeks | 1 year |
| Full-time | 32 | 26 | 5 | 19 |
| Part-time | 5 | 4 | 3 | 11 |
| Off work | 8 | 14 | 35 | 7 |
| Unemployed | 4 | 5 | 5 | 4 |
| Housewife[1] | 9 | 9 | 9 | 11 |
| Retired | 62 | 62 | 63 | 68 |
| *Total* | 120 | 120 | 120 | 120 |

[1] Includes housewives under the age of 65 years only

### Returning to work

In the first interviews, patients were asked whether they had been working before they had stoma surgery. In the second interviews patients were again asked about their employment status and, if they had returned to work, they were asked when they had done so.

The employment status of the sample at two months before surgery, at two weeks before surgery, at 10 weeks following surgery and one year later is given in Table 11.6.

The average time at which patients had returned to work was 24 weeks for ileostomates (8) and patients with urinary stomas (3) and 18 weeks for colostomates (19). Of those in full-time employment the majority were male (16). Ten of the 11 women who were working were employed part-time.

Undoubtedly, some of those who returned to work early were still unfit. For example, one man was working full-time as a farm labourer while having chemotherapy. Proximity of employment or self employment also appeared to enable patients to resume working sooner.

There was very little difference in the proportion of patients who returned to work between stoma nurse districts and non stoma nurse districts. Only one patient mentioned that he thought that his stoma was stigmatising and would be a barrier to obtaining employment. Fortunately, he had been able to discuss this with an established ostomate.

### Discussion

Taken as a whole, the findings from this study are encouraging in some respects and disappointing in others. For example, it is encouraging to see that, on average, patients appraised their lives more positively in comparison with before surgery and that the average level of social activities also appeared to have increased compared with before surgery. It is disappointing to find that almost one quarter of patients had been unable to come to terms with having a stoma although, as we have seen, this did not necessarily mean that they had curtailed their social activities or that the quality of life was any worse than before surgery.

At 10 weeks following surgery, patients' physical state, defined in terms of the extent and severity of symptoms, emerged as the single most important variable included in analysis. Physical state is still strongly related to patients' subjective appraisal of the quality of their lives, the degree to which they have resumed their social activities and their psychological adjustment one year after having surgery. Those patients who have a higher level of physical symptoms view their lives less positively and have increased their social activities to a lesser extent than those who have fewer symptoms. They are also more prone to anxiety or depression. Examination of the interview transcripts adds weight to this finding. Patients were either happier because their health had improved, they were free from pain, bladder or bowel management problems or they were no longer worried about their illness. On the other hand, many of those who were considerably less happy were socially restricted due to ill health or they were in pain. The notion that patients who are relatively free from symptoms will adapt more readily than those who are not is supported by these data.

One year after surgery, age appears to be less important, with regard to outcome, than at 10 weeks. It is related to patients' quality of life but, after controlling for physical state, age is unrelated to scores on the measure of social constraints or to scores on the measure of psychological adjustment. The hypothesis that adaptation to life with a stoma may be more difficult for older people is, therefore, supported only insofar as they view their lives less positively than before. It is not supported with regard to social constraints or to affective disorder.

The covariance analysis has shown that neither sex nor marital status bear a simple relationship with patient outcome. It would appear that unmarried males tend to do particularly well, viewing their lives more positively, increasing their social activities to a level greater than before surgery and being less prone to affective disorder. Unmarried males, whether single or widowed, tend to do far better than females who do not have the support of a spouse. In general, single or widowed females appraised their lives less positively than before surgery. Although they increased their social activities, relative to their level of activity before surgery, this was to a lesser extent than married women and was also to a lesser extent than men. Single or widowed females also seem to be more prone to affective disorder. The hypothesis that women may adapt less readily than men is therefore supported only with regard to those who do not have the support of a spouse. The hypothesis that married patients may adapt more readily than those who do not have the support of a spouse is supported for females but not for males.

Length of illness is strongly related to patients' self appraised quality of life and psychological adjustment. Those patients who had felt really ill for more than 3 months before surgery viewed their lives more positively than they had done before and were less prone to affective disorder. Outcome, with regard to social constraints, is somewhat more complex, inasmuch as married patients who had felt really ill for more than 3 months before surgery showed a large relative increase in social activities, whereas their unmarried counterparts showed little relative increase in social activities. The hypothesis that patients who had been ill for some time may adapt more readily to life with a stoma than those whose illness was of more rapid onset is, therefore, supported with regard to quality of life and psychological disorder. It is also supported with regard to social activities but only for those who have the support of a spouse.

Having access to a stoma care nurse is, for the most part, unrelated to patient outcome 1 year after surgery. In general, those patients who have access to a stoma care nurse are no more likely to appraise the quality of their lives more positively or resume their social activities to a greater extent than patients in districts which do not have the services of a stoma care nurse. Neither are they any less prone to anxiety or depression. The hypothesis that patients who have access to a stoma care nurse may adapt more readily than those who do not is not supported by these data. The possible reasons for this will be explored more fully in the next chapter. There is the somewhat puzzling finding that single or widowed ostomates in non stoma nurse districts increased their level of social activities to a much greater extent than single or widowed ostomates in stoma nurse districts. As unmarried males tend to do better than unmarried females it seems possible that this finding may be partially explained by the disproportionate distribution of the sexes. The unmarried group in stoma nurse districts comprised 16 females and 6 males whereas there were 9 females and 7 males in non stoma nurse districts. Had this been the complete explanation we would have expected a significant three-way interaction effect involving access to a stoma nurse, marital status and sex. This interaction effect did not reach significance. Therefore, it may be that this is largely a chance finding.

Patients were asked how many times they had seen a stoma care nurse during the past year. The average number of visits to patients in districts that had the services of a stoma care nurse was 4.8 but there were large variations in the number of visits made. The average number of visits made to patients who were anxious or depressed was 2.9. The range was from 0 to 13. The average number of visits made to patients who had not accepted their stoma was 3.75, the range was from 0 to 13. There was no relationship between patients' scores on the physical symptoms scale (PSS) and the number of visits made by stoma care nurses. These data would seem to suggest that the number of visits made by stoma care nurses was not based on any thorough patient assessment.

There is evidence that stoma care nurses took account of sex and marital status in the number of visits they made. For example the highest average number of visits was made to single or widowed females (7.6) and the lowest was made to single or widowed males (2.5). More visits were made, on average, to married women (6.8) than to married men (3.1). Thus, it would seem that stoma care nurses have correctly identified that single or widowed females may be at risk, but it would seem that the number of visits they make to patients is either based on a generalised view of patients, is in response to patient requests, or is based on some other criterion such as problems with appliances. A systematic approach to care based on a patient assessment which would identify those with physical or emotional problems appears to be lacking.

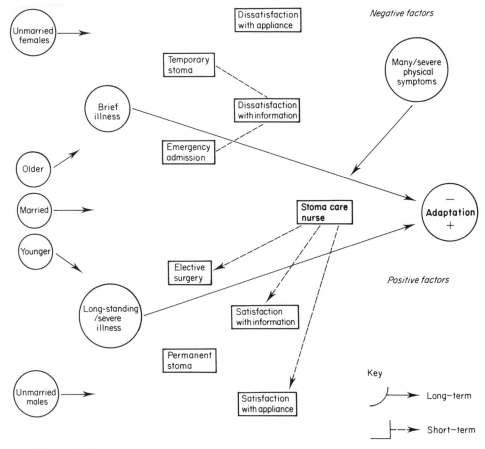

**Figure 11.5** Factors influencing adaptation to life with a stoma at 10 weeks and 1 year following surgery

It is now possible to amend the theoretical framework which was outlined in Chapter 1. Those factors which are related to patients' self assessed quality of life, level of social activity and psychological adjustment following stoma surgery are illustrated in Figure 11.5. Inter-relationships at 10 weeks following surgery are indicated by rectangles and broken lines. Factors related to outcome at both 10 weeks and 1 year following surgery are indicated by circles and solid lines.

In the next chapter, the possible reasons for these findings will be discussed and the results from this study will be compared with those from previous studies.

## Summary

One year after surgery the following factors were related to patients' subjective appraisal of their quality of life, social constraint or psychological adjustment:

(1) *Age*   Older patients appraised their lives significantly less positively than younger patients. Age was not related to social constraint or to psychological adjustment after controlling for physical state.

(2) *Physical state*   There was a very strong and negative relationship between the extent and severity of physical symptoms and patients' appraisal of the quality of their lives, social activity level and psychological adjustment.

(3) *Access to a stoma care nurse*   There was no significant difference with regard to quality of life or psychological adjustment between patients in stoma nurse districts and patients in other districts. Married patients in stoma nurse districts had lower levels of social constraint than married patients in non stoma nurse districts. However, the converse was true for those who did not have the support of a spouse.

(4) *Marital status × sex*   The self appraised quality of life and level of social activity was significantly greater for unmarried men than for married men but was lower for unmarried women than for married women. Married men were also more prone to affective disorder than those who were not married whereas there was little difference between married and unmarried women.

(5) *Length of illness before surgery*   Patients who had felt really ill for more than 3 months before surgery appraised the quality of their lives more positively and had lower levels of social constraint than those whose illness had been of shorter duration. Of those who had been ill for a longer period before surgery, married patients had lower levels of social constraint than those who were not married. Of those who had been ill for a shorter period before surgery married patients had higher levels of social constraint than those who were not married.

Additional analyses revealed that:

(6) The quality of life of patients who had ulcerative colitis or Crohn's disease was, on average, greatly improved compared with before surgery.

(7) Forty per cent of married ostomates said that they felt 'closer' to their spouse 1 year following surgery whereas 6% said that they felt further apart.

(8) Almost two-thirds of those who usually went away for a holiday had done so in the first year following surgery.

(9) On average, ileostomates and urostomates returned to work 24 weeks after surgery. Colostomates returned to work, on average, 18 weeks after surgery.

(10) Twenty-seven per cent of females and 19% of males reported that they were unable to accept their stoma 1 year after surgery.

# 12

# Clinical Nurse Specialists in Stoma Care?

### The findings in context

We have seen that, at 10 weeks following surgery, patients in stoma nurse districts were far better informed than patients in other districts. A greater proportion of patients in stoma nurse districts said that they had been told what to expect during their stay in hospital, they also had higher scores on the self-care information scale (SCIS) and appeared to be more satisfied with the information they had been given (Chapter 4). There was more family involvement in patient care in stoma nurse districts; a greater proportion of these patients said that they had had sufficient practice in changing their appliance before being discharged from hospital and more patients were independent of help in managing their appliance. At 10 weeks after surgery, we also saw that patients in stoma nurse districts were more satisfied with their appliance and that fewer of these patients had had at least one major accident with their appliance (Chapter 7). All these findings were statistically significant and they are clearly nursing outcomes.

Yet, despite these findings, we have also seen that patient adaptation to life with a stoma, defined in terms of self-assessed quality of life, social constraints and psychological adjustment, was not significantly different for patients in stoma nurse districts than for patients in districts which did not have the services of a stoma care nurse. Patients who had access to a stoma care nurse were no more likely to appraise the quality of their lives more positively or resume their social activities to a greater extent than patients in districts which did not have the services of a stoma care nurse either at 10 weeks after surgery or 1 year later. Does this imply that stoma care nurses are ineffective or are there other possible reasons for this lack of difference between the two groups of patients? For example, were the measures used in this study sufficiently sensitive to detect differences between the two groups of districts? Were the data contaminated in any way? Is adaptation to life with a stoma more of a medical than a nursing outcome? Were the stoma care nurses qualified and was their case load too heavy? Have the activities of stoma care nurses with regard to teaching, research and publications led to a greater awareness of the importance of stoma care generally? If this is so then the standard of care may have risen generally. Each of these possible explanations, any or all of which might contribute to a lack of difference in adaptation between the two groups, will now be examined in more detail.

## The measures

The measures employed in this study were specially designed for the purpose and they do highlight significant differences in relation to patient outcome with regard to factors other than having access to a stoma care nurse. For example, the bearing that length of illness before surgery, sex and marital status can have on patients' self assessment of quality of life, social activities and psychological adjustment have been discussed. The lack of difference in patient adaptation between the two sets of districts would not appear to be due to insensitivity of the measures.

## Contamination of data

At 10 weeks following surgery, 61% of patients in the 8 non stoma nurse districts had seen a company nurse/representative. Company nurses were operating in 6 of the 8 districts. In 5 of these districts they visited patients on the wards, in 2 districts they were siting the stomas and in 1 district the stoma clinic in the hospital was run by one of the appliance companies. Despite this degree of contamination, patients in stoma nurse districts were, as has been shown, more satisfied with their appliances. One year later 76% of these patients had seen a company nurse/representative. Indeed, a larger proportion of patients in non stoma nurse districts had changed to a different appliance since leaving hospital, and more than half of these had done so on the advice of a company nurse or, in a minority of cases, on the advice of a stoma care nurse from elsewhere. The difference in satisfaction with appliance found at 10 weeks after surgery was no longer evident. It would appear that there was considerable contamination of the data.

## Medical or nursing outcome?

'It is difficult to identify criteria solely attributable to nursing care, much less to one CNS's intervention. Cognitive, behavioural, and psychosocial variables can be more difficult to measure than health state but may often be the realm in which nursing makes its unique contribution to patient welfare.' (Hamric, 1983; p. 198)

An example of cognitive outcome, given by Hamric, is the increase in patient knowledge after institution of a teaching programme. An example of a psychosocial outcome would be improved social interaction or family understanding and participation in a patient's treatment. An example of a behavioural outcome might be patient compliance or adherence to a therapeutic regimen.

As we have already seen, some of these nursing outcomes were found in this study. Patients in stoma nurse districts had greater knowledge of self-care, family participation was greater and, although there was no significant difference between the two sets of districts, the average level of social activity at one year after surgery had risen in comparison with the level obtaining before surgery.

The biggest single factor relating to patient adaptation was the patient's physical state. In Chapter 4 we saw that, if those for whom an official diagnosis was not obtained are excluded, 70% of patients had a diagnosis of cancer. We have also seen that 16% of the sample died during that first year after surgery and some were too ill to be reinterviewed. The symptoms that some patients were experiencing on reinterview may have been heralding a recurrence of their disease. It may also be the case that a lurking fear of such a recurrence was the over-riding factor in determining the patient's quality of life and psychological adjustment. Similarly, as shown in the last chapter, the symptoms themselves served to reduce the level of patients' social activities.

To what extent, therefore, is the patient's physical state amenable to nursing interventions? The finding that the number of visits made by stoma care nurses did not relate to the patients' physical state needs to be interpreted with caution as it may be that those whom stoma care nurses did visit may have felt better as a result thus confounding the relationship. However, the lack of any formal patient assessment made by most of the stoma care nurses gives cause for concern and if further improvement in the standard of care for stoma patients is to be achieved a more detailed patient assessment is essential.

### The stoma care nurses

*Training*

There were 18 stoma care nurses in post in the 12 stoma nurse districts. Eleven of these had completed the full JBCNS course in stoma care. Two others, both of whom had responsibility for mastectomy patients, had done the short course. Five nurses, three of whom were assistants, were untrained in stoma care.

*Caseload*

Estimates of the number of new patients referred for each district each month ranged from 4 to 19 with a mean of 9.6. Estimates of the number of established ostomates seen each month in each district ranged from 20 to 70 with a mean of 50. Estimates of the distance travelled by each nurse each month ranged from 160 to 700 miles with an average of 352. Nurses in 9 of the 12 districts said that their caseload was about right, but in 3 districts it was described as too high. One of these nurses, who also had responsibility for mastectomy patients, said that she had about 10 new patients each month and also saw about 70 established ostomates travelling approximately 600 miles to do so.

## Teaching

All the stoma care nurses who were interviewed were involved in teaching the principles of stoma care to ward staff, all but one had given lectures to students in the school and many had given lectures to other staff including district nurses, pharmacists, GPs, dieticians, social workers and occupational therapists. In one district, the stoma care nurse arranged courses in stoma care.

## Research

All the nurses interviewed had been involved in clinical trials of new stoma care products and 4 had taken part in other research projects. Six had published articles on stoma care, and 11 out of the 12 nurses interviewed said that they read nursing journals, 8 of these recalling specific articles.

## A general rise in the standard of care?

Could these activities have been instrumental in raising the standard of care generally? The only way to shed light on this issue is to compare the findings from this study with those of previous studies of ostomates.

Grier et al (1964) report some decrease in social activities for 38% of a ·sample of 50 colostomates with an average time of 5.2 years after surgery. Druss et al (1969) took a retrospective look at 36 colostomates and report that there was a definite deterioration in social relationships in 72% of the group and that many of the patients were afraid of producing odour. George et al (1975) report that the social life of 22 out of 61 patients (36%) with permanent colostomy was curtailed following surgery. In this study, 19 of the 65 patients with permanent colostomies (29%) had a lower level of social activities than they had before surgery and when asked about odour only one patient said that this was often a problem.

The findings, with regard to holidays, also compare reasonably well with those from previous studies. For example, Eardley et al (1976) report a study of 76 colostomates who had had their stomas for varying lengths of time. They report that over half of the sample had been on holiday since the operation and that 18% had not been on holiday for stoma-related reasons, of which bag disposal was one. In this study, 55% of patients had taken a holiday during the first year following surgery and, as we have seen, others were also planning to do so. The percentage of patients who had not taken a holiday for stoma-related reasons is slightly lower than that obtained by Eardley et al.

Williams and Johnston (1983) carried out a study which involved 38 patients who had abdominoperineal excision of the rectum. The average time since surgery for these patients was 5.8 years. They report that 16 of the 26 patients (61.5%) who had taken an annual holiday preoperatively had taken a holiday since having surgery. The figures from this study are somewhat higher for APER patients in districts which had the services of a stoma care nurse. In the first year following surgery 69.4% of patients who usually took a holiday had done so and 16.7% said that they had not been away for stoma-related reasons. The figures for APER patients in non stoma nurse districts are not as good, 9 out of 18 patients had taken a holiday since having stoma surgery and 5 patients (27.8%) had not done so for stoma-related reasons.

In this study, 10 out of 19 patients (52.6%) who had permanent colostomies had returned to work, a further 3 had retired, 5 were 'off work' and 1 was unemployed. Williams and Johnston (1983) report that 6 of the 18 APER patients (33.3%) in their sample returned to work, 3 others retired and 9 patients could not work as a result of the operation. Devlin et al (1971) report that 24 out of 27 male colostomates changed their work habits following surgery and that the mean time off work was 31.1 weeks. In this study, the average time off work was 18 weeks for those colostomates who returned to work but 6 patients retired before being reinterviewed. It seems possible that some of the difference in the number who returned to work may be due to reduced employment opportunities generally and a trend towards earlier retirement. However the figures from this study compare favourably with those reported by Devlin et al and by Williams and Johnston.

Williams and Johnston (1983) also report that 12 of the 38 APER patients (32%) were found to be suffering from depressive illness. In this study, 12 of the 65 APER patients (18.4%) were assessed as depressed. Seven of the 41 APER patients in stoma nurse districts (17.1%) and 5 of the 18 APER patients in non stoma nurse districts (27.7%) were depressed. As differing lengths of time had elapsed since surgery and different measures were used these results are not strictly comparable. Nevertheless, there is a considerable difference between the figures produced by this study and those from the study by Williams and Johnston.

## Discussion

It would appear that failure to find a difference in patient adaptation between the two sets of districts is not due to insensitivity of the measures used.

However, two factors may have led to a reduction of potential differences between the two sets of districts. First, there is evidence of considerable contamination of the data due to the influx of company nurses or representatives into districts which did not have the services of an NHS stoma care nurse. Second, there is evidence that stoma care nurses were passing on their skills through teaching and through their efforts to publicise their work. These activities may have contributed to the overall rise in the standard of care for ostomates which is suggested when the findings from this study are compared to those of previous studies.

The strong relationship between patients' physical state and adaptation suggests that there are limits to the extent that nursing intervention may influence outcome at 1 year after surgery. There are strong indications that patient adaptation may be related to the disease process. In other words, adaptation may be as much as medical outcome as a nursing outcome.

From a social psychological point of view, it would seem that the outlook for patients following stoma surgery is less bleak than it used to be. Nevertheless, it would be a mistake to assume that this is due solely to the influence of stoma care nurses. For example, surgical techniques are improving. There have also been improvements in the range and types of appliance available to patients. Stoma care nurses have been involved in this through participation in trials of new or refined stoma care products. There is no means of knowing to what extent these factors have contributed to improving the outlook for patients who have to face life with a stoma.

A few years ago, it was suggested that the need for clinical nurse specialists would disappear as the new knowledge and skills that they demonstrated became part and parcel of everyday nursing activity (Tiffany, 1984). The turnover of nurses is such and the constant need to up-date our knowledge of stoma care products would seem to suggest that, for the foreseeable future, there will still be a need for the nurse with specialist knowledge of stoma care. How this knowledge is dispensed is another issue. In the next chapter, we will look at the factors influencing the appointment of clinical nurse specialists, the arguments for and against specialisation and the possible alternatives to the current structure of specialist nursing.

## Summary

(1) Despite the finding that, at 10 weeks following surgery, patients in stoma nurse districts were better informed and more satisfied with the information they had been given and with their appliances, there was no difference in adaptation between patients who had access to a stoma care nurse and those who did not.

(2) The possible reasons for this finding are discussed and the limitations of the study are clearly stated. One year after surgery, three-quarters of patients

in districts which did employ a stoma care nurse had been seen by a company nurse/representative.

(3)  In comparison with previous studies there is some evidence to suggest that the outlook for stoma patients has improved; the incidence of depression appears to be reduced and fewer patients appear to have curtailed their social activities.

# 13

# The Organisation of Care

On completion of the patient study, interviews were held with directors of nursing services, wards sisters and surgeons in the 20 districts included in the study. The aim of these interviews was to find out:

- the number and type of clinical nurse specialist posts and whether further posts were contemplated;
- what the incentives or disincentives were to the employment of clinical nurse specialists;
- the preferred role of stoma care nurses;
- the perceived contribution of stoma care nurses.

Although stoma care nurses were also interviewed in the 12 districts, the arguments presented in this chapter are mainly drawn from interviews with other members of staff.

## Clinical nurse specialist posts

The number and type of clinical nurse specialists employed in the 20 health districts is shown in Table 13.1. A total of 129 such posts was identified and, at the time of interview, consideration was being given to a further 25 posts. If these 20 districts are representative of all health districts, then the number of clinical nurse specialists has increased since 1982 when this study began and is still increasing. For example, one of the districts which did not have a stoma care nurse at the beginning of the study appointed such a nurse shortly before the staff interviews were carried out and three other districts were also contemplating such a post.

Table 13.1 also shows a shift in emphasis from 1982, with fewer specialists in infection control but more continence advisers, specialists in diabetes care, Macmillan nurses and liaison posts.

### Incentives and disincentives towards appointment

The major incentives towards the appointment of clinical nurse specialists throughout the 20 districts were:

**Table 13.1** The number and type of clinical nurse specialist posts in 20 randomly selected health districts

| Specialty | Stoma nurse districts n = 12 | | | Non stoma nurse districts n = 8 | | | All districts n = 20 | | |
|---|---|---|---|---|---|---|---|---|---|
| | Districts n | CNSs n | Under consideration n | Districts n | CNSs n | Under consideration n | Districts n | CNSs n | Under consideration n |
| Stoma care | 12 | 18 | – | 1 | 1 | 3 | 13 | 19 | 3 |
| Diabetes care | 9 | 12 | 2 | 5 | 5 | 1 | 14 | 17 | 3 |
| Geriatric liaison | 6 | 6 | 1 | 6 | 8 | 1 | 12 | 14 | 2 |
| Continence | 7 | 10 | 3 | 3 | 3 | 2 | 10 | 13 | 5 |
| Macmillan nurses | 3 | 4 | 2 | 3 | 8 | 1 | 6 | 12 | 3 |
| Paediatric liaison | 4 | 5 | – | 5 | 6 | 1 | 9 | 11 | 1 |
| Infection control | 6 | 6 | 1 | 1 | 1 | 1 | 7 | 7 | 2 |
| Community liaison | 2 | 2 | – | 2 | 5 | – | 4 | 7 | – |
| Terminal care | 2 | 4 | 2 | 2 | 2 | – | 4 | 6 | 2 |
| Mastectomy care | 4 | 4 | 1 | – | – | – | 4 | 4 | 1 |
| Chemotherapy | 2 | 3 | – | – | – | – | 2 | 3 | – |
| Community nursing | 1 | 2 | – | – | – | – | 1 | 2 | – |
| Leg ulcers | 1 | 2 | – | – | – | – | 1 | 2 | – |
| Pain control | – | – | – | 1 | 2 | – | 1 | 2 | – |
| Spinal injuries | 1 | 1 | – | – | – | – | 1 | 1 | – |
| Limb fitting | 1 | 1 | – | – | – | – | 1 | 1 | – |
| Handicapped | 1 | 1 | – | – | – | – | 1 | 1 | – |
| TB liaison | 1 | 1 | – | – | – | – | 1 | 1 | – |
| Cervical screening | 1 | 1 | – | – | – | – | 1 | 1 | – |
| Perinatal | 1 | 1 | – | – | – | – | 1 | 1 | – |
| Theatre | 1 | 1 | – | – | – | – | 1 | 1 | – |
| Child abuse | – | – | – | 1 | 1 | – | 1 | 1 | – |
| Stroke | – | – | – | 1 | 1 | – | 1 | 1 | – |
| Adult liaison | – | – | – | 1 | 1 | – | 1 | 1 | – |
| Genetic counselling | – | – | 1 | – | – | – | – | 1 | 1 |
| Haematology | – | – | 1 | – | – | – | – | – | 1 |
| Bereavement | – | – | 1 | – | – | – | – | – | 1 |
| *Total* | | 85 | 15 | | 44 | 10 | | 129 | 25 |

- patient need;
- cost effectiveness;
- caseload;
- pressure from consultants and from nursing staff;
- external sources of funding;
- factors specific to particular districts;
- dissatisfaction with the service offered by company nurses (with regard to stoma care nurses).

Similarly, lack of finance, insufficient caseload, factors specific to particular districts and satisfaction with the service provided by company nurses were disincentives towards the appointment of clinical nurse specialists.

### Patient need

Patient need was one of the main reasons given for the appointment of stoma care nurses. There were three main arguments based on the needs of patients. The first was that staff did not have enough time to counsel patients and give them the information they required before they were discharged from hospital:

'There just isn't enough time to go round, we don't spend nearly as much time as we ought to with these people. You have so many sick, heavy patients to look after. This is why I feel the stoma nurses really come into their own.' (Ward sister)

'The standard of care is borderline due to increased patient turnover and reduction in staff. I don't think I have enough staff in the ward at times to make it safe.' (Ward sister)

The second argument was that having stoma care nurses ensured that patients benefitted from continuity of care:

'Sometimes we don't even know that the patient is home until the GP gets a letter some 3 or 4 weeks later and sometimes the GP has had his letter and doesn't pass it over, so that there are some of these people that we are not aware of. There are a lot of people around who are suffering and I don't mean painfully, I mean miserably.' (Nurse manager)

Ward sisters often said that they had no idea about how stoma patients progressed after discharge from hospital:

'The problems start when they go home and are more isolated. You talk to your patients for a brief time and then they go out into the wide unknown and you don't know what happens after that.' (Ward sister)

The third argument was that nursing staff did not have the necessary expertise. For example:

'General nurses don't have time to gain expertise in all specialities or time to give to patients.' (Nurse manager)

'Community nurses are almost never well informed on this particular subject.'
(Nurse manager)

In specialties other than stoma care, patient need was more often the incentive
to appoint additional personnel. For example:

'The work grew so much, so our continence adviser now has an assistant.'
(Nurse manager)

### Cost effectiveness

In six districts it was said that the appointment of clinical nurse specialists in
diabetes care had been shown to be cost effective. Patients could be stabilised
at home and the number of admissions had been reduced. The changeover in
insulin was an additional incentive to the appointment of nurse specialists in
diabetes.

The cost effective argument was also made with regard to the appointment
of continence advisers, but in one district costs had increased following such
an appointment. In another district there had been an initial increase in costs
followed by a decrease in the long term:

'I think it gave a lot more patients satisfaction, which paid dividends in many
ways.' (Nurse manager, community)

The cost effective argument, in terms of reduced in-patient time, was also
made in respect of the appointment of a paediatric liaison nurse and a nurse
specialist in chemotherapy.

In two districts it was also stated that one of the incentives towards the
appointment of stoma care nurses had been the discovery of large amounts of
deteriorated stock and the lack of monitoring of the use of stoma care
products.

Six of the 8 districts that did not employ stoma care nurses said that lack of
finance was one of the reasons why stoma care nurses had not been appointed.

### Caseload

The size of the caseload in particular areas of care was also an incentive
towards the appointment of specialist nurses. For example, one district that
covered a large geographical area and had a large number of patients
undergoing stoma surgery was considering appointing a stoma care nurse. In
3 of the non stoma nurse districts the case load of stoma patients was said to be
rather small.

### Pressure from staff

Staff in several districts said that pressure from physicians was a factor in the
appointment of nurse specialists in diabetes. Complaints from GPs, consul-

tants and nursing staff to the effect that patients were not given adequate advice also provided an incentive to appoint stoma care nurses.

'The buffer zone of postoperative care and convalescence is being whittled away.' (Surgeon)

## External sources of funding

Two districts obtained funding in respect of regional and subregional specialities entailing cross boundary surgery and this enabled them to appoint nurse specialists in the relevant disciplines. External funding also appeared to be a strong influence on the appointment of Macmillan nurses.

## District factors

Factors specific to particular districts, such as the population structure, also influenced the appointment of nurse specialists. The size of the district and the number of outlying hospitals could be important. For example, one district had three general hospitals; two stoma care nurses were already in post but a third appointment was being considered at the time of these interviews. Other districts had several small neighbourhood hospitals and this increased the need for an efficient liaison scheme.

The size and geographical spread of two districts were also cited as reasons for not employing clinical nurse specialists in stoma care. For example:

'I think in a city it would be a much different situation but this is a large district and a nurse specialist would spend more time in the car than with the patients.' (Nurse manager)

## Company nurses

In three districts there was considerable dissatisfaction with the service provided by company nurses and this was said to be an incentive to appoint a stoma care nurse. For example, the director of nursing services (community) in one district that has since appointed a stoma care nurse, complained that conflicting advice was being given to patients by company nurses from different firms:

'Each tended to push their own product when what we wanted was the right product for the patient irrespective of the brand.'

The complaint that company nurses tended to push their own product and that they had insufficient time or were not always available was repeated in two other districts, one of which was also considering the appointment of a stoma care nurse.

However, satisfaction with the service provided by company nurses was a disincentive towards the appointment of stoma care nurses in two other districts in which these nurses gave a full service, visiting the wards, siting stomas, teaching staff and not restricting patients to one particular brand of appliance:

> 'She is very good and she will teach the nurses as well. She is an extra special person. I mean she has an obligation to . . . but we keep all sorts of appliances on the ward and she will use those if it is better for the patient.' (Ward sister)

In another district, the company nurse ran an out-patient stoma clinic in conjunction with a ward sister who had herself completed a full course in stoma care.

### Attitudes of staff

As has been shown, pressure from staff was sometimes an incentive towards the appointment of specialist nurses, but hostility or negative attitudes towards the concept of specialist nursing were also major disincentives. Such attitudes were more commonly, but not exclusively, held by staff in districts which did not employ stoma care nurses. Negative attitudes were based on four main arguments.

The first argument is based on the premise that the development of specialist nursing detracts from the role of the generalist. Specialism in nursing results in a lack of commitment to patients by other staff who may abdicate from the caring role or, in respect of the ward sister, from the teaching role. This leads to a diminishing of the skills of the nurse generalist. The following quotations were taken from the transcripts of interviews with staff mainly in non stoma nurse districts.

> 'If you have a problem and you know that the stoma nurse is going to come, then you will leave it to her.' (Ward sister)

> 'All the sisters will, inevitably, leave the teaching to the specialist nurse.' (Nurse manager)

> 'The district nurse will take to just perhaps a "popping in" role and will not give actual care.' (Nurse manager, community)

> 'The stoma nurse just comes to look at the stoma. They don't see the whole patient.' (Nurse manager)

However, negative attitudes were occasionally expressed in stoma nurse districts also:

> 'One wonders whether or not you are denying or depriving nurses of that richness of experience which we have.' (Nurse manager)

> 'I consider that specialisation leads to de-skilling both in the individual specialist and in the generalist. The generalist says, "That is not my job" and fails to maintain her level of knowledge or her practical skills and the individual specialist, because she knows more and more about less and less, is less adaptable and less able to progress.' (Nurse manager—stoma nurse district)

The second argument is that increasing specialisation in nursing leads to the fragmentation of care:

'You get a multiplication of communications with the increased number of people that are going in to provide a service for that patient.' (Nurse manager, community)

'Care is becoming fragmented. I feel sorry for the district nurses. Now that they have a recognised training we must be very careful.' (Stoma care nurse).

The third argument is that specialism in nursing does not provide career opportunities:

'They are in a professional cul de sac.' (Nurse manager)

'Where does the specialist nurse go after she has been doing her job for 5 years?' (Nurse manager)

The fourth and final strand to these arguments is that nurse specialisms are based on a medical model of care:

'Nursing specialties also worry me because they are not truly nursing specialties. In the main, we follow medical specialties but they are often developed to support, not even medical specialties, but individual consultants. Sometimes the creation of a specialist post is a "get-out" for ineffective management which has failed to ensure the delivery of services to those who need them. There is very rarely any attempt to really quantify the need before they create it.' (Nurse manager)

This particular allegation appeared to be unfounded. These interviews revealed that studies to estimate patient need or to review an existing service were being carried out in seven districts.

### The preferred role of stoma care nurses

Nurse management, ward sisters and surgeons were also asked how they saw the role of clinical nurse specialists and stoma care nurses in particular. Staff in one district, where attitudes to specialisation were particularly hostile, did not comment.

Two major components emerged in these discussions. The first was that the clinical nurse specialist should act as a resource for other members of staff. This viewpoint was spontaneously expressed in all 12 stoma nurse districts and in 6 of the 8 non stoma nurse districts. It was a commonly held view among nurse managers in the community, for example:

'It would be important that she liaised closely with the district nurse prior to any surgery. Then be with them throughout the period in the hospital and early discharge but then become the resource for that patient through the district nurse.' (Nurse manager)

The second component was that of teaching other members of staff. This was also mentioned in all 12 stoma nurse districts and in 6 of the 8 non stoma nurse districts.

> 'They could detract if they took over and didn't pass on any knowledge.' (Ward sister)

Staff in 5 districts suggested that clinical nurse specialists should act as consultants when other staff are faced by difficult patient problems. Direct patient care was spontaneously mentioned by staff in 7 districts, 2 of which said that this should be limited to in-patients. Coordination or liaison was specified in 3 districts, patient counselling in 2 districts, improving or updating the service in 2 districts and research in 2 districts.

Staff in one non stoma nurse district linked these components. For example, the stoma care nurse should give direct care to in-patients and liaise with community staff, thus allowing early discharge. Subsequently, she should act as a resource for staff.

Staff in another non stoma nurse district related the role to the spread of the district. In a large health district the teaching and resource components were of paramount importance in view of the distance that would have to be covered to give direct patient care in the community.

### The perceived benefits of clinical nurse specialists in stoma care

*Surgeons*

Thirteen surgeons were interviewed, 8 of whom were in stoma nurse districts. Six of the 8 surgeons in stoma nurse districts said that they approved the appointment of stoma care nurses, the other 2 expressed guarded approval. One of the 5 surgeons interviewed in non stoma nurse districts expressed extreme disapproval of the idea of specialist nurses in stoma care:

> 'The medical profession has given up on the nursing profession. The nurses can go their own way and we will see where they end up.'

Another was cautious in his comments:

> 'There is a real risk of highly-trained young ladies doing highly technical things in the office with sophisticated cleaners looking after the patients.'

*Ward sisters*

Ward sisters were asked whether they felt that stoma nurses were of benefit or whether they detracted from their role. Eleven of the 12 ward sisters in stoma nurse districts said that patient care was improved or that patients were 'better off'. Indeed, one ward sister suggested that the care given to ostomates was better than that given to other groups of patients. There were three aspects to this improved patient care. The first was the expertise of the stoma care nurse.

For example, five ward sisters spontaneously mentioned that the stoma care nurse had extended their knowledge:

'They have taught me everything I know. Twenty years ago when I started my training, stomas to me were things like raw skin—distressed patients and frightened nurses. The nurses had little knowledge and the patients had no knowledge.' (Ward sister)

The second aspect was that the stoma care nurse had the time to listen and to counsel patients and the third was that she could provide for continuity of care after discharge.

There was one dissenting voice from a ward sister in a district in which an untrained stoma care nurse was employed:

'She's not relieved us much at all. She should spend more time teaching patients and students.'

This ward sister also said that the appliances used were 'out of date'.

Ward sisters in non stoma nurse districts were also enthusiastic about the possible benefits from stoma care nurses. Five viewed stoma nurses as having additional expertise, 4 said that they would be 'up to date', 4 mentioned that there was insufficient time, 2 said that patients would benefit and 2 mentioned continuity of care. Only 1 of these ward sisters felt that any benefits were in theory only.

*Community nurse managers*

Interviews with community nurse managers in stoma nurse districts revealed a lesser degree of enthusiasm. Three said that care was improved, others said that district nurses were not involved unless the patient had other needs such as a wound problem. It also emerged that patients were not always referred and that sometimes district nurses were not even informed when patients were discharged. Of the 8 community nurse managers in non stoma nurse districts 3 were dissatisfied with the care given to ostomates and felt that this might be improved with specialist input. Three reported antagonism on the part of district nurses who felt that this would detract from their role.

An alternative system

One district had devised a different system of providing care:

'We have sisters with specialist interests rather than clinical nurse specialists. We support them to attend various courses and study days and to have an overall view of all patients within their specialty within the hospital.' (Director of nursing services)

Thus, one ward sister had a special interest in stoma care and had completed the full course. She attended out-patient sessions, sited stomas, taught nurses in training and was used as a resource by other staff:

> 'She gives advice and teaches so that other people are available and are capable of doing it.' (Director of nursing services)

However, an interview with this ward sister revealed that she didn't feel that she had sufficient time to give the extra care that patients needed:

> 'It is the time element again. I am sure a full-time stoma therapist could do a lot more.'

A similar system was operating in the community:

> 'We really felt that we should not limit the role of the district nursing sister. If we did have specialist nurses in every specialty we would limit the district nursing sisters to mundane jobs and we would lose staff. Our district nursing sisters teach within their own teams and they also deal with the patients themselves and we feel that this gives more specialist patient care to every patient. We are not actually against specialist nurses.'

In this district the stomal clinic was run by one of the appliance companies.


### Discussion and conclusion

Given the incentives outlined above, it is hardly surprising that there has been an increase in the appointment of clinical nurse specialists. Perhaps the most powerful argument for specialist knowledge is that of patient need, but cost effectiveness, access to additional funding and staff attitudes may be more powerful incentives.

The attitudes of staff were clearly divided but there was a distinct trend for more positive attitudes on the part of hospital staff than for community staff. All but one of the ward sisters in stoma nurse districts felt that patients received better care, many felt that their knowledge had improved and, as has been shown, the stoma care nurses in this study were extensively involved in teaching the principles of stoma care to staff on the wards. Therefore, it would appear that the alleged detraction from the role of the generalist does not occur within the hospital setting. This study does provide evidence which suggests that district nurses make fewer visits to patients in those districts which employ stoma care nurses. The Cumberlege Report (DHSS, 1986) states that:

> 'Specialist nurses working from a hospital base sometimes provide nursing care and advice in people's homes without prior consultation with district nurses or health visitors, causing confusion for the client and unnecessary friction between hospital and community services.' (p. 11)

The interviews with community nurse managers indicate that such friction may occur in some health districts. However, the allegation that stoma care nurses detract from the role of district nurses would be upheld only if district nurses gave care that is comparable to that given by stoma care nurses. Evidence of the lack of knowledge, given by some nurse managers in the community, suggests that this is not so. Moreover, the interviews with patients 1 year after surgery provide no evidence that patients in non stoma nurse districts consult with district nurses when they have problems that they wish to discuss.

There is an interesting anomaly with regard to the service provided by company nurses. It would appear that negative attitudes towards clinical nurse specialists do not prevent some districts from making use of the services of company nurses. This would seem to add a whole new dimension to the specialist/generalist argument. The input of these nurses/representatives is such that we need to examine the implications rather carefully. The following points are relevant:

(1) All the stoma care nurses interviewed had been involved in clinical trials of new or refined stoma care products, one third had taken part in other research projects and one half had published articles on stoma care. Will company nurses do likewise and if they do will they achieve the same degree of objectivity?

(2) NHS stoma care nurses typically stock at least three makes of appliance and inform patients about the different types of appliance available. Only 15% of ostomates subsequently changed to a different brand of appliance during the first year following surgery. Thus, the majority of patients remained faithful to the make of appliance they first use. Discussions with ward sisters in this study suggest that not all company nurses give patients this initial choice, indeed one such nurse removed other brands of appliance from the ward:

'Well . . . is our contract so we just use . . . appliances.' (Ward sister)

(3) In this study, patients with temporary stomas fared less well initially than patients with permanent stomas. Their knowledge of self-care was less than that of permanent ostomates in districts which did not have the services of a stoma care nurse. Will company nurses have the same incentive to care for temporary ostomates when this group has limited market potential?

(4) By the end of the first year following surgery three-quarters of the patients in districts which did not have the services of a stoma care nurse had seen a company nurse. However, the proportion of patients who cited the NHS stoma care nurse as having been of most help to them since discharge was far greater than the proportion of patients who had seen and who cited a company nurse.

(5) Manufacturers compete for the market by improving the quality of their products. The stoma care nurses provide this incentive. The market is dominated by three brands of appliance. The presence of so many manufac-

turers' representatives at conferences held by the Stoma Care Forum leaves one in no doubt as to the importance of the market in stoma care products. One rather disconcerting finding in this study was that very few of the stoma care nurses we interviewed were accountable for their budget. If they were, then manufacturers would have to compete with regard to costs as well as quality thus achieving a cost effective service in the long term.

These considerations are not presented as an argument for increasing the number of nurse specialists in stoma care. There is certainly an argument for nursing care to be given by someone with special knowledge or with access to special knowledge. How that care is dispensed is a complex issue.

A horizontal structure in line with the recommendations of the Cumberlege Report (DHSS, 1986), in which nurses with special knowledge are used as a resource by other members of staff, may be more appropriate to nursing. Such a structure might be particularly appropriate in districts in which the caseload of patients with particular technical or care needs is small or in districts which have a large geographical spread. Such a system would need to be carefully monitored to ensure that patients received the care that they required.

One of the arguments against the current structure is that specialist nursing is based on a medical model of care. If the present structure were the most appropriate and effective way of providing care then this argument would be of academic interest. However, within the medical model care is given to specific patient groups identified on the basis of disease and/or medical treatment. It is, in effect, a compartmentalised vertical structure. It may be that this model is not the most appropriate for all health districts or for all nurse specialties. Moreover, accusations that the present structure leads to the de-skilling of nurse specialists themselves merit special consideration. The present form of specialisation within nursing does not appear to have provided the clinical career structure which was originally envisaged.

A nursing model would imply that patient groups would be identified by a common need for care. The components of care, over and above the technical aspects, can be similar for many of the nurse specialties. For example, many of the different nurse specialists need to have counselling and teaching skills. They all need to know how to make a thorough assessment of the patient's care requirements.

If specialisation in nursing is based on a medical model of care, then so too is the education of nurse specialists. If education for nurse specialists were to be based on a nursing model, it would focus on the common components of care and not on patient groups. A core curriculum could include courses on counselling techniques, teaching skills and patient assessment. Additional topics relating to technical aspects for particular groups of patients could be covered in short courses. Such as approach would obviate the need to cover the same ground again should a nurse wish to acquire knowledge applicable to a different patient group. It would also be less expensive and time consuming.

For example, a nurse with specialist knowledge in stoma care who had completed the basic course would only require a brief education relating to the technical aspects to qualify as a nurse with specialist knowledge of the care of mastectomy patients. It would also be easier for a nurse to extend or to update her technical knowledge.

In the introduction to this study we said that a major development in nursing, such as the big increase in the number of nurses specialising in various areas of care, should not rest on an assumption that the service to patients will be improved. This study was designed to test this assumption in respect of one area of care—that given to patients who have had stoma surgery.

Despite extensive contamination of data due to the influx of company nurses/representatives into districts which did not employ stoma care nurses, the study provides strong evidence that nursing outcomes are better in those districts which employ stoma care nurses. There is also some evidence to suggest that the outlook for patients undergoing stoma surgery is less bleak than it used to be. There may be room for further improvement and this may hinge upon a thorough patient assessment of nursing care requirements.

The findings from this study are not prescriptive. In this final chapter we have examined the organisation of care and clearly there is no universal recipe. We now need to recognise that the specialist/generalist argument is naive. If stoma patients benefit from specialist care then efforts should be made to provide such care but the way in which it is provided is an organisational issue which only management can decide at a local level. Moreover, we cannot comment on other nurse specialties. A second research project is focused on the work of nurses who specialise in the care of diabetic patients, but that is another story.

# References

Abrams J S (1984) *Abdominal Stomas.* Boston: John Wright.

Abrams R D and Finesinger J (1953) Guilt reactions in patients with cancer. *Cancer,* **6:** 474–482.

Aldridge M C and Sim A J W (1986) Colonoscopy findings in symptomatic patients without X-ray evidence of colonic neoplasms. *The Lancet,* **ii,** 833–834.

Barney M (1978) Emotional aspects of colostomy and ileostomy. *Psychosomatics,* **19(4):** 214–218.

Barney M and Perlman A (1971) Emotional response to ileostomy and colostomy in patients over the age of 50. *Geriatrics,* **25(6):** 113–118.

Beadle C (1981) Caring for a patient with a stoma. *Geriatric Medicine,* **11:** 59–65.

Black P (1985) Stoma care, 1. Selecting a site. *Nursing Mirror,* **161(9):** 22–24.

Bond S (1983) Nurses' communication with cancer patients. In: *Nursing Research,* ed. Wilson-Barnett J, pp. 57–80. Chichester: John Wiley.

Brady N (1984) Nursing Times editorial: Lack of education on stoma problems. *Nursing Times,* **80:** 6.

Brady N (1985) The theory of nursing and the future role of the stoma care nurse. In: *The Future Role of Stoma Care Nursing.* Report of a seminar held in Copenhagen. Oxford: Medical Education Services Ltd.

Breckman B E (1977) Care of the stoma patient. *Nursing Mirror,* supplement, **145(13):** i–iv.

Breckman B (1979) Keep the customer satisfied. *Journal of Community Nursing,* **3(2):** 4–7.

Breckman B E (1979b) Role of the nurse specialist in stoma care. *Journal of Human Nutrition,* **33:** 383–387.

Breckman B (1980) The Stoma and the Patient. *Nursing Mirror,* Supplement, **150(4):** i–xiii.

Brewin T B (1977) The cancer patient: communication and morale. *British Medical Journal,* **ii:** 1623–1627.

Broadwell D C (1983) Nursing specialization: the enterostomal therapy nurse. *Occupational Health Nursing,* **45:** 15–19.

Bromley B (1980) Applying Orem's self care theory in enterostomal therapy. *American Journal of Nursing,* **LXXX:** 245–249.

Brown J S (1984) Sigmoidoscopy in general practice. *The Practitioner,* **228:** 837–839.

Castledine G (1982) *The Role and Function of Clinical Nurse Specialists in England and Wales.* Unpublished MSc thesis, University of Manchester.

Chandler J G and Evans B P (1978) Colostomy prolapse. *Surgery,* **84(5):** 577–582.

Chisholm E M, Dombal F T and DeGiles G R (1985) Validation of a self administered questionnaire to elicit gastrointestinal symptoms. *British Medical Journal,* **290:** 1795–1796.

Cohen F (1975) Psychological preparation, coping and recovery from surgery. In: *Health Psychology,* eds Stone G C, Cohen F and Adler N E. London: Jossey-Bass.

Cohen F and Lazarus R S (1973) Active coping processes, coping dispositions and recovery from surgery. *Psychosomatic Medicine,* **35:** 375–389.

Cohen F and Lazarus R S (1982) Coping with the stresses of illness. In: *Health Psychology*, eds Stone G C, Cohen F and Adler N E. London: Jossey-Bass.

Cunningham M E (1969) *A Demographic Survey of Ostomates*. Unpublished MA thesis, Kent State University.

DHSS (1980) *The Provision of Stoma Care*. London: HMSO.

DHSS (1986) *Neighbourhood Nursing—A Focus for Care*. Report of the Community Nursing Review (The Cumberlege Report). London: HMSO.

Devlin H B (1976a) Management of a colostomy and its complications. In: *Modern Stoma Care*, ed. Walker F C. London: Churchill Livingstone.

Devlin H B (1976b) The structure and function of a colostomy. In: *Modern Stoma Care*, ed. Walker F C, pp. 41–56. London: Churchill Livingstone.

Devlin H B (1984) Stomas and stoma care. In: *Textbook of Gastroenterology*, eds Bouchier I A D, Allan R N, Hodgson H J F and Keighley M R B. London: Baillière Tindall.

Devlin B (1985) Second opinion, *Health and Social Services Journal*, part 1, p. 82.

Devlin H B, Plant J A and Griffin M. (1971) Aftermath of surgery for anorectal cancer. *British Medical Journal*, **iii;** 413–418.

Donaldson R J (1976) Community support for the stomatist. In: *Modern Stoma Care*, ed. Walker F C. London: Churchill Livingstone.

Druss R G, O'Connor J F and Stern L O (1969) Psychologic response to colectomy. *Archives of General Psychiatry*, **20:** 419–427.

Druss R G, O'Connor J F, Prudden J F and Stern L O (1968) *Archives of General Psychiatry* **18:** 53–59.

Eardley (1979) Stoma care. *The Practitioner*, **222:** 264–266.

Eardley A, George W D, Davis F, Schofield P F, Wilson M C, Wakefield J and Sellwood R A (1976) Colostomy: the consequences of surgery. *Clinical Oncology*, **2:** 277–283.

Elcoat C (1986) *Stoma Care Nursing*. London: Baillière Tindall.

Elian M and Dean G (1985) To tell or not to tell the diagnosis of multiple sclerosis. *The Lancet*, **ii:** 27–28.

Engstrom B (1984) The patients' need for information during hospital stay. *International Journal of Nursing Studies*, **21(2):** 113–130.

Feighner J P, Robins E, Guze S B, Woodruff R A, Winokur E and Munoz R (1972) Diagnostic criteria for use in psychiatric research. *Archives of General Psychiatry*, **26:** 57–63.

Fleming J (1984) Bags of choice. *Senior Nurse*, **1(23):** 1009.

Fuller J H S (1984) Ano-rectal bleeding. *The Practitioner*, **228:** 825–828.

Gazzard B G and Dawson A M (1978) Diets and stomas. In: *Intestinal Stomas*, ed. Todd I P, pp. 133–149. London: W B Saunders.

George W D, Eardley A, Davis F N and Schofield P F (1975) Problems of permanent colostomy. *Gut*, **16:** 408.

Gilholme Herbst K and Humphrey C (1980) Hearing impairment and mental state in the elderly living at home. *British Medical Journal* **281:** 903–905.

Gillon R (1985) Paternalism and medical ethics. *British Medical Journal* **290(i):** 1971–1972.

Grier W R N, Syarse A and Localio S A (1964) Evaluation of colonic stoma management without irrigations. *Surgery, Gynecology and Obstetrics*, **118:** 1234–1422.

Hall J N (1974) Inter rater reliability of ward rating scales. *British Journal of Psychiatry*, **125:** 248–255.

Haan N G (1982) Psychosocial meanings of unfavourable medical forecasts. In: *Health Psychology*, eds Stone G C, Cohen F and Adler N E. pp. 113–140. London: Jossey-Bass.

Hamric A B (1983) A model for developing evaluation strategies. In: *The Clinical Nurse Specialist in Theory and Practice*, eds Hamric A B and Spross J, pp. 187–206. London: Grune and Stratton.

Hopkins A (1985) Telling patients the diagnosis. *The Lancet*, **ii:** 214.

Hutchinson G H and Weston P M T (1984) Progress in colorectal cancer. *The Practitioner*, **228:** 771.

Irving M (1982) Ileostomy, In: *Stomas*, eds. Brookes B N, Jeter K F and Todd I P, pp. 237–246. London: W B Saunders.

Jackson B S (1975) Colostomates: the mosaic of stress and implied care. *Australian Nurses Journal*, **4(10):** 24–27.

Jackson B S (1980) The growing role of nurses in enterostomal therapy. In: *Seminars in Oncology*, vol. VII, no. 1, ed. Yarbro J W, pp. 48–55.

Janis I L and Rodin J (1982) Attribution, control and decision making: social psychology and health care. In: *Health Psychology*, eds. Stone G C, Cohen F and Adler N E. London: Jossey-Bass.

Kay D W K, Beamish P and Roth M (1964) Old age mental disorders in Newcastle upon Tyne. *British Journal of Psychiatry*, **110:** 146–158.

Kelly M P (1985) Loss and grief reactions as responses to surgery. *Journal of Advanced Nursing*, **10:** 517–525.

Kelly M P (1986) The subjective experience of chronic disease: some implications for the management of ulcerative colitis. *Journal of Chronic Diseases*, **39(8):** 653–666.

Kelly M P (1987) Managing radical surgery: notes from the patient's viewpoint. *Gut*, **28(1):** 81–87.

Kretschmer K P (1978) *The Intestinal Stoma*. Philadelphia: W B Saunders.

Langer E J (1983) *The Psychology of Control*. London: Sage.

Lerner J, Harsh J, Eisenstat T E (1980) Why pre-op stoma planning is a must. *R N Magazine*, **75(8):** 48–51.

Locker D and Dunt D (1978) Theoretical and methodological issues in sociological studies of consumer satisfaction with medical care. *Social Science and Medicine*, **12:** 283–297.

MacDonald L D, Anderson H R and Bennet A E (1982) *Cancer Patients in the Community: Outcomes of Care and Quality of Survival in Rectal Cancer*. Department of Clinical Epidemiology and Social Medicine, St George's Hospital Medical School, London.

MacDonald L D and Anderson H R (1984) Stigma in patients with rectal cancer: a community study. *Journal of Epidemiology and Community Health*, **38:** 284–290.

Maguire P, Lee E G, Bevington D J, Kuchemann C S, Crabtree R J and Cornell C E (1978) Psychiatric problems in the first year after mastectomy. *British Medical Journal*, **15(ii):** 963–965.

McIntosh J (1974) Processes of communication, information seeking and control associated with cancer: a selective review of the literature. *Social Science and Medicine*, **8:** 167–187.

McKenna S E (1979) A new lease of life. *Nursing Times*, **75(8):** 320–323.

Meaney M (1985) The role of the stomatherapist. *World of Irish Nursing*, **4(4):** 5–6.

Mitchell A (1980) Patients' views on stoma care. *Nursing Mirror*, **151:** 38–41.

Morrison J (1978) Rehabilitation of the ostomate. *Australian Nurses Journal*, **8(2):** 46–48.

Morrison J (1981) Suitable only for loners. *Australian Nurses Journal*, **10(9):** 36–37.

Morrow, L (1976) Psychological problems following ileostomy and colostomy. *Mount Sinai Journal of Medicine*, **43(4):** 368–370.

Nichols S, Koch E, Lallemand R C, Heald R J, Izzard L, Machin D and Mullee M A (1986) Randomised trial of compliance with screening for colorectal cancer. *British Medical Journal*, **293:** 107–110.

Nordstrom G and Hulten L (1983) Loop ileostomy as an alternative to transverse loop colostomy. *Journal of Enterostomal Therapy*, **10**: 92–94.

Northover J M A (1984) Colorectal cancer—today and tomorrow. *The Practitioner*, **228**: 569–572.

Orbach C E and Tallent N (1965) Modification of perceived body and of body concepts. *Archives of General Psychiatry*, **12**: 126–135.

Parkes C M (1972) *Bereavement: Studies of Grief in Adult Life*. London: Tavistock.

Plant J A (1976) Rehabilitation: nursing care and the role of the stoma nurse. In: *Modern Stoma Care*, ed. Walker F C, pp. 12–24. London: Churchill Livingstone.

Prudden J F (1971) Psychological problems following ileostomy and colostomy. *Cancer*, **28**: 236–238.

Reeves K (1984) More than sticking on bags. *Senior Nurse*, **1(23)**: 19.

Saunders B (1976) Clinical nurse consultant in stoma care. *Nursing Mirror*, **142**: 54–58.

Seligman M E P (1975) *Helplessness: On Depression Development and Death*. San Francisco: Freeman.

Sredl D and Wilhite M (1980) The enterostomal therapist—a new breed of nurse. *Supervisor Nurse*, **1(1)**: 51–52.

Stockley A (1982) Stoma care services: in hospital. In: *Stomas*, eds Jeter K F and Todd I P. pp. 373–376. London: W B Saunders.

Stringer M S (1985) *The Future Role of Stoma Care Nursing*. Report of a Seminar held in Copenhagen. Oxford: Medical Education Services Ltd.

Sutherland A M, Orbach C E, Dyk R B and Bard M (1952) The psychological impact of cancer and cancer surgery. *Cancer*, **5(5)**: 857–872.

Swaffield L (1979) Finding the problems. *Nursing Times*, Community Outlook, **4**: 66–75.

Tabachnick B G and Fidell L S (1983) *Using Multivariate Analysis*. New York: Harper and Row.

Tiffany B (1984) The splinter effect. *Nursing Times*, **80**: 33.

Trainor M A (1982) Acceptance of ostomy and the visitor role in a self help group for ostomy patients. *Nursing Research*, **31(2)**: 102–106.

Vowles K D J (1978) After colostomy, the problems begin. *Modern Geriatrics*, **8(1)**: 26–27.

Walker F C (1976) Ileostomy. In: *Modern Stoma Care*, ed. Walker F C, pp. 71–83. London: Churchill Livingstone.

Williams N S and Johnston D (1980) Prospective controlled trial comparing colostomy irrigation with 'spontaneous-action' method. *British Medical Journal*, **ii**: 107–109.

Williams N S and Johnston D (1983) The quality of life after rectal excision for low rectal cancer. *British Journal of Surgery*, **70**: 460–462.

Wilson D (1981) Changing the body's image. *Nursing Mirror*, **152**: 38–40.

Wilson Barnett J and Osbourne J (1983) Studies evaluating patient teaching: implications for practice. *International Journal of Nursing Studies*, **20(1)**: 33–44.

Wing J K, Cooper J E and Sartorious N (1974) *Measurement and Classification of Psychiatric Symptoms*. Cambridge: Cambridge University Press.

Young Wood R and Watson P G (1977) People with temporary colostomies. *The Canadian Nurse*, **73**: 28–30.

# Appendix

**Completely Confidential**

The Royal College of Nursing of the United Kingdom
The Daphne Heald Research and Development Unit
**Stoma Care Interview Schedule**

| | Case number |
|---|---|
| | |

*Var. no.*

Date ................................................ Completed by ................................

Patient code ................................... District ☐☐ 1

Group ☐ 2

| | | | Var. no. |
|---|---|---|---|
| 3. Age | | | ☐☐ 3 |
| 4. Sex | | | ☐ 4 |
| 5. Marital Status | | | ☐ 5 |
| 6. Religion | | | ☐ 6 |

| 7–9. Education/Employment | 2 months before stoma | 2 weeks before stoma | Now | |
|---|---|---|---|---|
| In full-time education | 1 | 1 | 1 | |
| In part-time education | 2 | 2 | 2 | ☐☐ 7 |
| In full-time employment | 3 | 3 | 3 | |
| In part-time employment | 4 | 4 | 4 | |
| Off school indefinitely | 5 | 5 | 5 | ☐☐ 8 |
| Off work indefinitely | 6 | 6 | 6 | |
| Unemployed | 7 | 7 | 7 | |
| Retired (including housewives over 65) | 10 | 10 | 10 | ☐☐ 9 |
| Housewife | 11 | 11 | 11 | |

**If patient has returned to education/employment post-operatively:**

10. When did you return to work? ........................................... ☐☐ 10

11. Date of operation ......... Number of weeks postoperative ......... ☐☐ 11

12. Date of discharge ......... Number of days in hospital ............... ☐☐ 12

13. Convalescent home? ..... Number of days in convalescent
                      home ......................................................... ☐☐ 13

14. How long did you feel really ill before your operation? ......... ☐☐☐ 14

15. Type of stoma:
    Ileostomy           1
    Colostomy         2
    Urostomy          3                       ☐ 15
    More than one stoma  4

☐T   Why did you have the operation?

☐T   What did they tell you about the operation?

16. Is your stoma a permanent one?
    Yes          1
    No           2                       ☐ 16
    Don't know  9

    (Check—have they taken your 'bottom' away?)

17.  | Circle site of stoma on diagram |

                                             ☐ 17

18. Who decided where the stoma was to be sited? ................... ☐☐ 18

19. Can you see your stoma easily?
    Yes         1
    No          2                       ☐ 19
    Don't know  9

20. When did you first look at your stoma?
    In hospital       1
    After discharge   2                    ☐  20
    Have not looked  3
    Don't know      9

**If patient has seen his/her stoma:**

T   How did you feel when you first saw your stoma?

21. Were you reluctant to look at it at first?
    Yes          1
    No          2                    ☐  21
    Don't know  9

**If patient has not seen his/her stoma:**

T   Is there any reason why you haven't looked at it yet?

22. While you were in hospital were you given any written
    information, a booklet for example?
    Yes         1
    No         2                    ☐  22
    Don't know  9

**If patient was given written information:**

23. Who gave you this information?  ..................  ☐☐  23

24. Were you told what would happen during your stay in
    hospital?
    Yes         1
    No         2                    ☐  24
    Don't know  9

**If patient was told what would happen:**

    What were you told?  ..................

25. Who told you this?  ..................  ☐☐  25

26. Was there anything else that you would like to have been told
    about?
T   Yes         1
    No         2                    ☐  26
    Don't know  9

Did any of the following people come to see you in hospital?

| | Visited | | | Not visited | | | |
| --- | --- | --- | --- | --- | --- | --- | --- |
| | helpful | neither helpful nor unhelpful | not helpful | would have liked visit | not needed | DK | NA |
| 27. Stoma nurse | 5 | 4 | 3 | 2 | 1 | 9 | 8 | ☐ 27 |
| 28. Company nurse | 5 | 4 | 3 | 2 | 1 | 9 | 8 | ☐ 28 |
| 29. Social worker | 5 | 4 | 3 | 2 | 1 | 9 | 8 | ☐ 29 |
| 30. GP | 5 | 4 | 3 | 2 | 1 | 9 | 8 | ☐ 30 |
| 31. Stoma visitor | 5 | 4 | 3 | 2 | 1 | 9 | 8 | ☐ 31 |
| 32. Other | 5 | 4 | 3 | 2 | 1 | 9 | 8 | ☐ 32 |

**Now I would like to ask you about information you were given about what to expect when you were discharged from hospital:**

| Were you told about? | Who gave information? | |
| --- | --- | --- |
| 33. How to clean your stoma | ☐☐ | 33 |
| 34. The different types of appliance available | ☐☐ | 34 |
| 35. How to change your appliance | ☐☐ | 35 |
| 36. How often to change your appliance | ☐☐ | 36 |
| 37. How to dispose of used appliances | ☐☐ | 37 |
| 38. How to obtain a further supply | ☐☐ | 38 |
| 39. What to do if any problems arose | ☐☐ | 39 |
| 40. Eating and drinking | ☐☐ | 40 |
| 41. How to remove adhesive | ☐☐ | 41 |
| 42. Shrinkage of stoma | ☐☐ | 42 |
| 43. Leakage | ☐☐ | 43 |
| 44. Self-help groups | ☐☐ | 44 |
| Number of items | ☐☐ | 45 |

46. Have you joined any self-help groups?
    Yes                    1
    No, but interested     2          ☐ 46
    No, not interested     3

47. Was anyone in your family given any information about the care of your stoma?

| | |
|---|---|
| Yes | 1 |
| No, would have liked | 2 |
| No, family didn't want | 3 |
| No, patient didn't want this | 4 |
| Not applicable | 8 |
| Don't know | 9 |

☐ 47

48. Did you have any practice in changing your appliance prior to discharge?

| | |
|---|---|
| Yes, sufficient | 1 |
| Yes, insufficient | 2 |
| No | 3 |
| Don't know | 9 |

☐ 48

Since you came home have any of these people been to see you?

| | Visited | | | Not visited | | | |
|---|---|---|---|---|---|---|---|
| | helpful | neither helpful nor unhelpful | not helpful | would have liked visit | not needed | DK | NA |
| 49. Stoma nurse | 5 | 4 | 3 | 2 | 1 | 9 | 8 | ☐ 49 |
| 50. Company nurse | 5 | 4 | 3 | 2 | 1 | 9 | 8 | ☐ 50 |
| 51. Social worker | 5 | 4 | 3 | 2 | 1 | 9 | 8 | ☐ 51 |
| 52. GP | 5 | 4 | 3 | 2 | 1 | 9 | 8 | ☐ 52 |
| 53. Stoma visitor | 5 | 4 | 3 | 2 | 1 | 9 | 8 | ☐ 53 |
| 54. District nurse | 5 | 4 | 3 | 2 | 1 | 9 | 8 | ☐ 54 |
| 55. Health visitor | 5 | 4 | 3 | 2 | 1 | 9 | 8 | ☐ 55 |
| 56. Other | 5 | 4 | 3 | 2 | 1 | 9 | 8 | ☐ 56 |

Since you came home have you visited:

| | visited helpful | visited not helpful | not visited | don't know | | Reason for visit | |
|---|---|---|---|---|---|---|---|
| 57. Stoma clinic (nurse) | 3 | 2 | 1 | 9 | 58 | ☐☐☐ | 57–58 |
| 59. GP surgery | 3 | 2 | 1 | 9 | 60 | ☐☐☐ | 59–60 |
| 61. OPD | 3 | 2 | 1 | 9 | 62 | ☐☐☐ | 61–62 |

63. Have you been readmitted to hospital?
    Yes   1
    No    2                                                    ☐   63

64. For what reason? .............................................................................
T   .............................................................................   ☐   64


**Now I would like to ask you a few questions about your appliance:**

65. What make of appliance are you using? ........................   ☐☐☐   65

66. Who fixes your appliance?
    Self              1
    Parent            2
    Spouse            3
    Other relative    4                                        ☐   66
    District nurse    5
    Stoma nurse       6
    Other             7


**If help is needed:**

67. Who usually helps?
    Parent            2
    Spouse            3
    Other relative    4
    District nurse    5                                        ☐   67
    Stoma nurse       6
    Other             7
    Not applicable    8

68. Why is this? .............................................................................
T   .............................................................................   ☐☐   68

69. How long does it usually take to change the bag? (minutes)   ☐☐   69

70. How often is the bag usually changed?
    More than once a day   1
    Once a day             2
    Every 2 or 3 days      3                                   ☐   70
    Every 4 days or more   4


**Two-piece appliance only:**

71. How long does it usually take to change the bag and flange
    together? (minutes)                                        ☐☐   71

72. How often is the flange usually changed?
    More than once a day    1
    Once a day    2
    Every 2 or 3 days    3
    Every 4 days or more    4
    Not applicable    8

☐ 72

73. How often were you told to change the flange?
    More than once a day    1
    Once a day    2
    Every 2 or 3 days    3
    Every 4 days or more    4
    Not applicable    8

☐ 73

74. Is the bag (and flange) easy or difficult to remove?
    Very easy    1
    Reasonably so    2
    Very difficult    3

☐ 74

75. Do you have any problems with leakage?
    Yes    3
    Occasional accident    2
    No    1

☐ 75

76. Does the adhesive part either wrinkle or peel off during wear?
    Yes    3
    Sometimes    2
    No    1

☐ 76

77. Does the skin become irritated?
    Yes    3
    Sometimes    2
    No    1

☐ 77

78. Does the appliance get in the way when you change position?
    Yes    3
    Sometimes    2
    No    1

☐ 78

**Total** ☐☐ 79

80. Have you modified your appliance in any way?
    Yes    1
    No    2

☐ 80

**If yes**

81. In what way?......................................................................................... ☐ 81

**Show card**

82. How comfortable is your appliance?

Not at all         Extremely
comfortable        comfortable

☐☐☐ 82

83. How easy is your appliance to change?

| Extremely | Extremely | |
| difficult | easy | 83 |

84. How confident are you in your appliance?

| Not at all | Extremely | |
| confident | confident | 84 |

85. All things considered, how satisfactory is your appliance?

| Not at all | Extremely | |
| satisfactory | satisfactory | 85 |

**Total** 86

87. Have you changed the type of appliance you use since you left
hospital?
   Yes   1
   No    2                                                                87

**If patient has changed his/her appliance:**

88. Why did you change? ................................................................
T                   ................................................................                    88

89. Who recommended the change? ........................................   89

90. Have you had any problems in obtaining a further supply of
appliance?
   Yes   1
   No    2                                                                91

**If yes**

T   What kind of problems? ................................................................

91. Has your stoma altered in shape since you left hospital?
(specify)
   Yes, smaller          1
   Yes, other change     2
   No                    3                                               91
   Don't know            9

**(Show card)**

|  | Have you experienced? How often | Do you still have this now? How often |  |
|---|---|---|---|
| 92. Pain |  |  | 93 |
| 94. Backache |  |  | 95 |
| 96. Flatus |  |  | 97 |
| 98. Bad smells |  |  | 99 |
| 100. Noisy stoma |  |  | 101 |
| 102. Discolouration of stoma |  |  | 103 |
| 104. Sensation of rectal fullness (APER only) |  |  | 105 |
| 106. Urinary infection |  |  | 107 |
| 108. Incontinence |  |  | 109 |
| 110. Constipation |  |  | 111 |
| 112. Diarrhoea |  |  | 113 |
| 114. Prolapse |  |  | 115 |
| 116. Retraction of stoma |  |  | 117 |
| 118. Narrowing (stenosis) of stoma |  |  | 119 |
| 120. Abdominal wound infection |  |  | 121 |
| 122. Abdominal wound hernia |  |  | 123 |
| 124. Problems with perineal wound |  |  | 125 |
| 126. Fatigue |  |  | 127 |
| 128. Ulceration of stoma |  |  | 129 |
| 130. Infection (stoma) |  |  | 131 |
| 132. Slight bleeding (stoma) |  |  | 133 |
| 134. Severe bleeding (stoma) |  |  | 135 |
| 136. Obstruction (blockage) |  |  | 137 |
| 138. Sweating |  |  | 139 |
| 140. Indigestion |  |  | 141 |
| 142. Nausea |  |  | 143 |
| 144. Vomiting |  |  | 145 |
| 146. Discharge |  |  | 147 |
| 148. Other (specify) |  |  | 149 |
|  | **Total** |  | 150 |
|  | **Diff. Scores** |  | 151 |

152. Are there any foods which you used to eat before you had
     surgery but which you don't eat now?
     Yes           1
     No            2                                               ☐ 152
     Don't know    9

**If yes**

     What are these foods? ..................................................................................

153. Are there any foods which you eat now but which you didn't
     eat before you had surgery?
     Yes           1
     No            2                                               ☐ 153
     Don't know    9

**If yes**

     What are these foods? ..................................................................................

154. Is the change in your diet because of your operation or for some
     other reason?
     Operation        1
     Other reason     2
     Not applicable   8                                            ☐ 154
     Don't know       9

**I would like to ask you about some everyday activities:**

⊤    Is there anything that you used to do before you had surgery that is more
     difficult for you to do now? (Probes: bathing, dressing, cleaning,
     shopping, laundry, cooking, driving, using public transport, bending,
     stretching, carrying, climbing stairs, walking, cutting toenails, gardening)

     ..................................................................................................................

⊤    Is there anything that you used to enjoy doing that you feel you can't do
     now?

     ..................................................................................................................

**Show card**

Before you had surgery
how often did you:            Before      Now      Comments

155. Visit friends                                           □□  155–156
157. Have friends in                                         □□  157–158
159. Go to clubs/pubs                                        □□  159–160
161. Go to church                                            □□  161–162
163. Participate in a
     sport (social)                                          □□  163–164
165. Go out for a meal                                       □□  165–166
167. Go out for a cup
     of tea                                                  □□  167–168
169. Use public transport                                    □□  169–170
171. Go to parties                                           □□  171–172
173. Go to evening classes                                   □□  173–174
175. Go to the cinema/theatre                                □□  175–176
177. Take part in hobbies
     (social, other than sport)                              □□  177–178
179. Other (specify)                                         □□  179–180

                              **Total**      □□  181
                              **Diff**           182
                              **Mean diff**  □□□  183

Overall, would you say that you enjoy life more or less than you did before
you had surgery?

184.            Enjoy very        Enjoy very
                much less         much more                   □□□  184

Overall, would you say that you are more or less active than before you
had surgery?

185.            Very much         Very much
                less active       more active                 □□□  185

Overall, would you say that you are more or less happy than before you
had surgery?

186.            Very much         Very much
                less happy        more happy                  □□□  186

                              **Total**  □□□  187

**If more/less happy:**

T̲   Why? ....................................................................................................................................

188. Was any one person particularly helpful while you were in hospital?

   ................................................................................................................   ☐☐  188

189. Who has been the most helpful person since you were discharged from hospital?

   ................................................................................................................   ☐☐  189

190. If you needed some help with your stoma whom would you contact?
   (If no response, probe—spouse, etc.)

   ................................................................................................................   ☐☐  190

   Overall, what do you think has been the main problem for you?

T̲   ....................................................................................................................................

   Apart from the actual operation, is there anything about your stay in hospital which particularly stands out in your memory?

T̲   ....................................................................................................................................

**Psychological adjustment (present state examination)**

I would like to get some idea about how you have been feeling over the last *4 weeks*

that is, since ................................................................

*First, can I ask you how you have been feeling physically*, apart from what you have already told me?

Rate subject's own *subjective* evaluation of present physical health:
   0=feels physically very well
   1=has no particular complaint but does not say positively feels fit
   2=feels unwell but not seriously incapacitated
   3=feels seriously incapacitated by physical illness

                                     Physical health (1)   ☐

*Have you worried a lot during the past 4 weeks?*

What do you worry about?

What is it like when you worry?

What sort of state of mind do you get into?

Do unpleasant thoughts constantly go round and round in your mind?

Can you stop them by turning your attention to something else?

Rate *worrying*, i.e. frequent painful thoughts which cannot be stopped and out of proportion to the subject worried about:

1 = symptom definitely present during past 4 weeks, but of moderate intensity,
or intense less than 50% of the time
2 = symptom intense more than 50% of the month

Worry (2) ☐

*Over the last 4 weeks, have you had any headaches?*

What kind?

Rate only tension pains, for example 'band around the head', 'pressure'
'tightness in scalp', 'ache in back of neck':
1 = symptom definitely present during past month but of moderate clinical
intensity, or intense less than 50% of the time
2 = symptom clinically intense more than 50% of past month

Tension pains (3) ☐

*Have you been getting exhausted and worn out during the day or evening, even
when you have not been working very hard?*

In what way?

Rate tiredness or exhaustion—do not include tiredness due to influenza, etc:
1 = only moderate form of symptom (tiredness) present, or intense form
(exhaustion) less than 50% of the time
2 = intense form of symptom (exhaustion) present more than 50% of past
month

Tired/exhausted (4) ☐

*Have you had difficulty relaxing during the past month?*

Do your muscles feel tensed up?

Rate muscular tension—do *not* include a subjective feeling of nervous tension
which is rated later:
1 = symptom definitely present during past month but of moderate clinical
intensity or intense less than 50% of the time
2 = symptom clinically intense more than 50% of past month

Muscular tension (5) ☐

*Do you often feel on edge or keyed-up or mentally tense or strained?*

Do you generally suffer from your nerves?

Do you suffer from nervous exhaustion?

Rate *subjective* feeling of nervous tension:
1 = symptom definitely present during past month, but of moderate intensity,
or intense less than 50% of the time
2 = intense form of symptom present more than 50% of past month

Nervous tension (6) ☐

*Have there been any times lately when you have been very anxious or
frightened?*

What was this like?

Did your heart beat fast? Ask for other autonomic symptoms.

How often in the past month?

Rate free-floating autonomic anxiety (exclude if due to delusions; exclude if purely situational)
    1 = symptom definitely present, with autonomic accompaniment, during past month, but of moderate clinical intensity, or intense less than 50% of the time
    2 = symptom clinically intense more than 50% of the time
                    Free-floating autonomic anxiety (7) ☐

*Have you had the feeling that something terrible might happen?*

That some disaster might occur but you are not sure what?

Have you been anxious about getting up in the morning because you are afraid to face the day?

What did it feel like?

Rate anxious foreboding with autonomic accompaniments:
    1 = symptom definitely present, with autonomic accompaniment, during past month, but of moderate clinical intensity, or intense less than 50% of the time
    2 = symptom clinically intense more than 50% of the time
            Anxious foreboding with autonomic accompaniments (8) ☐

*Have you had times when you felt shaky or your heart pounded, or you felt sweaty, and you simply had to do something about it?*

What was it like?

What was happening at the time?

How often during the past month?

Rate panic attacks with autonomic symptoms (a panic attack is intolerable anxiety leading to some action to end it, e.g. leaving a bus, phoning husband at work, going to see a neighbour, etc.:
    1 = one to four panic attacks during month
    2 = panic attacks 5 times or more
              Panic attacks with autonomic symptoms (9) ☐

*Do you tend to get anxious in certain situations, such as travelling, or being alone, or being in a lift?*

What situations? How often during the past month?

### Checklist

Crowds (shop, street, cinema, theatre, church)

Going out alone, being at home alone

Enclosed spaces (hairdresser, phone booth, tunnel)

Open spaces (bridges)

Travelling (buses, cars, trains)

Rate situational autonomic anxiety
    1 = has not been in such situations during past month, but aware that anxiety would have been present if the situation had occurred

2=situation has occurred during past month and patient did feel anxious
                    Situational autonomic anxiety (10)   ☐

*Do you keep reasonably cheerful or have you been very depressed or
low-spirited recently*

Have you cried at all?

When did you last really enjoy doing anything?

Rate depressed mood (N.B. when rating clinical severity of depression
remember that deeply depressed people may not necessarily cry):
  1=only moderately depressed during past month, or deep depression for less
    than 50% of time, and tending to vary in intensity
  2=deeply depressed for more than 50% of past month, and tending to be
    unvarying in intensity
                    Depressed mood (11)   ☐

*How do you see the future?*

Has life seemed quite hopeless?

Can you see any future?

Have you given up or does there still seem some reason for trying?

Rate hopelessness on subject's own view at present:
  1=hopelessness of moderate intensity but still some degree of hope for the
    future (irrespective of time during month)
  2=intense form of symptom (has given up hope altogether)
                    Hopelessness (12)   ☐

*Have you ever felt that life wasn't worth living?*

Did you ever feel like ending it all?

What did you think you might do?

Did you actually try?

Rate suicidal plans or acts:
  1=deliberately considered suicide (not just a fleeting thought) but made no
    attempt
  2=suicidal attempt but subject's life never likely to be in serious danger,
    except unintentionally
  3=suicidal attempt apparently designed to end in death (i.e. accidental
    discovery or inefficient means)   .
                    Suicidal plans or acts (13)   ☐

*Have you been much more irritable than usual recently?*

How do you show it?

Do you keep it to yourself, or shout, or hit people?

How do you normally show your irritation?

Rate irritability:
  1=keeps irritation to herself
  2=shows anger by shouting or quarrelling

3=shows anger by hitting people, throwing or breaking things
                                                    Irritability (14)  ☐

*What has your appetite been like over the last 3 months?*

Have you lost any weight recently?

Rate weight loss due to poor appetite providing not due to physical illness:
    1 =less than 7 lb (3.2 kg)
    2=7 lb or more
                                                    Loss of weight (15)  ☐

*Have you had any trouble getting off to sleep during the past month?*

How long do you lie awake?

Do you take sleeping tablets? Do they help?

Rate delayed sleep (must have occurred at least 10 or more nights over last month:
    1 =1 hour or more delay (irrespective of sleeping tablets)
    2=2 hours or more delay (irrespective of sleeping tablets)
                                                    Delayed sleep (16)  ☐

*Do you wake early in the morning?*

Rate early waking (one hour before usual):
    1 =1 hour or more before ordinary time
    2=2 hours or more before ordinary time
    In either case must have occurred 10 or more nights in last month
                                                    Early waking (17)  ☐

*Has there been any change in your physical relationship with your husband, that is, your interest in sex?*

How has it changed?

Rate loss of libido:
    1 =definite lessening of interest and performance
    2=almost total loss or total loss of libido
                                                    Loss of libido (18)  ☐

Were you given any information about this?

Are there any other comments you would like to make?

Would you consent to a further short interview at a later date?

**Thank you for your help**

# Index

Page numbers in **bold** refer to figures and tables